CONTENTS

WITHDRAWN FROM STOCK

KT-429-543

FOREWORD

Robin Berzin, M.D.

For a long time our definition of health has pivoted on the external. How we look gets more airtime than how we feel. And yet we know that when it comes to the myriad of chronic conditions so many of us battle in the modern age – from weight gain to uncomfortable digestive issues, chronic fatigue to hormonal imbalances and more – it is truly what is on the inside that counts.

In the past few years new research has shed light on how gut health defines overall health. We know that the microbiome – the trillions of bacteria that live inside our bodies – not only help to digest our food but also impact countless other functions.

We know that different bacteria populations are associated with weight gain versus weight loss and that the health of your microbiome can dictate how fast your metabolism runs, how often you get sick, and even how happy (or sad) you regularly feel.

Yes, the medications we take and the foods we eat define the composition of these populations. But beyond that, we now have proof that certain lifestyle factors – including environmental toxins, stressors, hydration, and activity level – can affect not only how our gut behaves and how we digest our food, but also which bacteria in our systems live and die.

All of this together is what is known as the science of 'systems biology' – the idea that the body is an interconnected matrix, constantly in flux in response to stimuli from both inside and outside. The systems biology approach helps us understand why 'eat this, not that' and calorie counting regimens don't work – our bodies are much more complicated, and much more intelligent, than that.

Still, with all this groundbreaking research, the key question is, how do we take what science is telling us and make it relevant to our daily lives? In my 10-plus years as a physician working on the cutting edge of medicine, what I've seen missing – and the reason why so many people are still struggling with stubborn weight and gut issues – is a truly inside-to-outside perspective that makes sense with a fast-paced, modern lifestyle.

This is what makes *Reset Your Gut* special. In this book, Robyn Youkilis has taken her experience with the hundreds of people she has coached one on one and married it with the latest science. She's created a step-by-step food and life plan for shedding weight and finding optimal health by focusing first on your insides – your gut.

This approach is the only one I see sustainably work for people.

Let Robyn guide you to achieving your personal goals and beyond in her caring and thoughtful way. Be patient and go at your own speed. And as you'll learn in this book, listen to your gut. Remember, the key to success is truly already within you.

INTRODUCTION

I've struggled with my weight for most of my life. I've had good days and bad days that were based entirely on how tight my jeans felt when I pulled them on. Despite being a bestselling author, appearing as a wellness expert on national television shows, helping hundreds of clients through my health-coaching practice (Your Healthiest You) and reaching even more on social media, I'm just like millions of other women out there who look in the mirror and think, 'My bum's too big!'

Everyone has their own journey, their quest to feeling vibrant and happy in their body. For me, it began when, in a desperate attempt to lose weight, I finally stopped eating junky diet foods and started eating real foods and focussing on truly nourishing my gut.

I'm now – well into my thirties and having had a baby – at my lightest weight and the most comfortable I've ever been in my body. But it wasn't that long ago that I was totally frustrated with doing 'all the right things' without seeing the right results.

I know I'm not alone. The average adult gains about half a kilo of weight each year from age twenty-five on. This fact, along with a slowing metabolism, increased stress levels and a whole host of other reasons is why we find ourselves with weight to lose at some point in our adult lives. But, as easy as it is to pack on the kilos, you can instead choose to listen to your body, drop the distracting mental chatter and optimise your digestion. This is your gut's secret to finding your best body no matter what stage you're at in your life.

I hear success stories all the time from my inspiring clients and friends who have followed my approach to gut health and weight loss. People from Brooklyn to LA, Australia to the UK tell me my approach has helped them understand their bodies and feel good after a lifetime of diet drama and belly woes. In my first book, *Go with Your Gut*, I explained digestive health in a way that allowed readers to connect with their own gut instincts, learn how to make food choices from a place of inner wisdom, banish bloat and leverage the amazing power of the simple act of chewing. I have women all over the world making more home-cooked meals, slowing down and discovering the foods and practices that help them feel their best.

Here are just a few of the stories I've received from my readers and clients:

> With Robyn's help, I learned how to listen to my body by thinking about what kind of food would feel good rather than running on autopilot. While I used to make the same breakfast every day, I began to check in: Did I want one egg or two? Gluten-free toast or leftover roasted vegetables? Did I even need coffee? Did I want some avocado, and how much? I also started prepping food for my day, to ensure I would have good things to turn to rather than the vending machine or an open bag of crisps. I no longer feel guilt about food or think about specific foods as being 'bad' or 'good'. Instead, I eat what my body wants and needs, as well as what I know will make me feel like my best self in the long run. — AMY

I'm now eating breakfast, drinking tons of infused water, loving my gut-friendly smoothies and actually enjoying cauliflower! Robyn was right – good digestion is the key to everything! Better skin, mental clarity and more! Thanks for teaching me how to take better care of myself! — PRISHA

Participating in Robyn's virtual Chewing Challenge has taught me to stop inhaling my food and slow down during meals. Now that I chew my food completely, not only do I enjoy eating even more, I've realised that I actually don't need as much food as I thought I did! As a result, my belly has become tighter, I feel so much more comfortable in my clothes, and I'm loving the pure joy of not having to constantly adjust my trousers over my bloated belly! — ALEXANDRA

One of my clients even bragged to me that her husband now eats sauerkraut and kale. That's what I consider real success!

While these transformations illustrate what's possible for anyone with a little information and motivation, what I heard more and more from my readers, clients and community was the need for a plan; specifically, a weight-loss plan.

WHAT THIS BOOK IS ABOUT

This book will show you how stubborn weight can melt away when you tune into your gut and learn to heal from the inside out. Beyond that, it will show you how to feel comfortable, confident and energised in this home that is your body.

What I see out in the holistic health world is a lot of dancing around the topic of weight loss. I see a lot of quick-fix approaches that address the symptoms (i.e. belly bloat and weight gain) but not the underlying issues. What's missing is an understanding of why it's so hard to lose the weight and keep it off.

Luckily for you, this book is not another diet book. I won't be assigning grapefruit-only days or cheat days. I'm here to give you straight health talk as someone who is truly passionate about wellness and has spent her life studying health and nutrition. After decades of self-motivated study and an official health-coaching certification from the Institute for Integrative Nutrition, I started my coaching practice, Your Healthiest You, almost a decade ago. In my life, I've worn a lot of hats – and a lot of clothing sizes, too, probably just like you.

MY DEFINITION OF WEIGHT

Let's first talk about weight and what it really means. It's more than just a number on the scales. Even though I weigh only about five kilos less than I did ten years ago, I look a hundred times better now. That's because ten years ago, I was carrying around a considerable amount of 'emotional weight'.

♦ I was desperately searching for how to 'get it right' with my food.

♦ I was partying way too much and looking for love in all the wrong places – from the newest leader of the band in the world's skinniest jeans to celebrities who were up to no good.

♦ I was unfulfilled and unhappy in my jobs.

♦ I felt lost in what I was doing with my life and was too afraid to show up when I had glimpses of a 'higher calling'.

♦ I had no flow or rhythm in my day.

♦ I was carrying credit-card debt and quickly depleting the savings I had worked so hard to build.

So what do I mean by 'weight' (and weight loss) in the context of this book?

Weight is a feeling in your body.

> **A DESIRE TO LOSE WEIGHT IS A SIGN THAT WE WANT SOMETHING TO BE DIFFERENT IN OUR BODIES, BUT EVEN MORE SO, IN OUR LIVES.**

For example:

Are you feeling guilty about your food choices, mainly because you think you should 'know better'?

Does the anxiety from your high-pressure job show up as daily indigestion or heartburn?

Do you rely on your glass of wine at the end of the day to unwind?

Do you giggle at the idea of 'eating your feelings', but know this is exactly what you're doing with your nightly snacking ritual?

Do you feel like you never have enough (in the bank, in your wardrobe, in the pantry)?

Are you feeling unsettled in your life, even though you can't put your finger on exactly what needs to change?

What you need is a physical weight-loss plan, in addition to a plan that will help you shed emotional weight. You've got to learn to let go of what's not serving you, so you can live your healthiest life and feel amazing.

If your goal is to be lighter in body, belly and spirit, then this book will guide you there. When I eat according to the Go with Your Gut Weight-loss Formula, I feel nourished and full. I'm not worried about calories and my clothes fit just fine. When I don't eat this way, my digestion declines (leading to bloating and problems pooping), and the old restrictive Robyn diet-brain – 'eat this, don't eat that' – rears its ugly head.

For example, I was on holiday with my family in upstate New York and I forgot my sauerkraut (OMG, how COULD I?). I wasn't making my famous yogurt power parfaits for breakfast. I wasn't structuring my plates like I teach in this book. This was fine for a day or two, but by the fourth day, my husband had to literally rip the third serving of Carvel ice-cream cake out of my hands.

I share this story to highlight how what you eat affects the delicate balance of bacteria in your digestive tract. When the bacteria in your gut is off kilter, you start to crave more sweets and you feel exhausted and down on yourself. You can't make solid choices from this place.

The weight-loss philosophy I teach in this book is simple and easy to follow. Your body wants you to feel good, and the best way to reach your natural weight is to keep your gut flora happy and balance the other parts of life that 'weigh' you down. Together, these two forces will have you looking and feeling fabulous.

WHAT MOST DIETS ARE MISSING

Have you been on a diet 'forever' but still have 'those last X kilos' to lose? Do you feel like you stay on top of all the wellness trends, but there's still something you're missing – a secret trick that everyone knows except you? Or do you feel as though you're doing all the right things but your body isn't responding? Why can't you just lose the weight?

◆ Your gut's not working.

When I say 'gut' here, I mean both your physical gut and your gut instincts, your intuition. If your gut isn't working, nothing works. The weight stays on your belly and hips like that annoying ex-boyfriend you can't stop thinking about. But it goes beyond that. You feel stuck in your life. You're doing okay, but you feel as though you're not really nailing it – your diet, your workout plan, or even what you chose to wear today. After reading this book and following the Go with Your Gut Weight Loss Formula, everything will start to fall into place.

◆ The way you digest your food is the way you 'digest' your life.

We'll cover emotional weight loss along with the physical and practical components to powerfully move you forward to your ultimate vision of you. If you've been on the weight-loss train for years (or decades), you've probably noticed that even though you've lost weight in the past, it likely didn't feel (or look) the way you hoped it would. It's only when you're willing to look at all the parts of you – body, mind and heart – that you'll finally feel the lightness you've been looking for on the scales.

THE GUT HEALTH–WEIGHT LOSS CONNECTION

When it comes to physical gut health, you may be wondering what exactly digestion has to do with weight loss. 'Robyn, I get that gut health may help with annoying issues like bloating and gas, but how does that relate to that extra weight I can't seem to lose?'

The answer is: *everything*.

Yes, healing your gut can help you get rid of embarrassing digestive issues, but it can do so much more than that. There are three main reasons why gut health is directly linked to reaching your ideal weight:

1 A healthy gut better absorbs nutrients from the food you are eating.

2 A healthy gut knows exactly what you need to feel your best. It's your connection to your intuition, your unique gift that directs your best choices in life.

3 A healthy gut means a happier you. This is the brain-gut connection I can't wait to share more about.

I will break down the science and the key components of 'how' and 'why' behind these points in chapter one.

REBECCA'S STORY

My client Rebecca shifted much more than just her weight using the same principles I'm teaching in this book. When she came to me, she was a busy executive at a big tech company in San Francisco, stressed out and burnt out from eating the 'right' foods in the wrong way.

Rebecca was already having salads for lunch and going to the gym regularly when she came to me, but her life and body still weren't clicking. Working in tech, she had way too many options at lunchtime, with a lavish spread of delicious, free food always available. Rebecca followed the Go with Your Gut Weight Loss Formula and learnt to breathe properly and actually chew her food.

Rebecca started using my simple 123 Food Freedom Tool (which you'll learn on page 67) at lunchtime in the crazy cafeteria. She would visit the cloakroom before going to the cafeteria and simply stand in the cubicle taking a few deep breaths, one hand on her heart and one on her belly. She'd ask herself what she really wanted to eat and what would feel great. By plugging this tool into her routine, she started making simple, nourishing choices that follow the Good Gut Rule of Five (see pages 26–7). Rather than stressing and agonising over food decisions like she used to, she started finding it easier to choose the option she knew was best for her.

Rebecca also began cooking for herself more often. As a single woman with a full-time job, she found the meal-prep tips 'life-changing'. When she stocked her fridge and pantry the Go with Your Gut way, she stopped reaching for the office snacks every afternoon and stopped ordering takeaways every night. Get this: Rebecca used to travel internationally for work at least eight times a year and she would take her own meals to eat on her business-class flights! Keeping her digestion regular by taking her own food to eat while on the road was key to her transformation.

Since restoring her gut through cooking, chewing and breathing, Rebecca feels relaxed, light and free around food. She recently switched jobs to a company more aligned with her lifestyle, is studying to become a health coach and started teaching yoga classes. How cool is that?! Wondering how you can make some of the shifts Rebecca made? Well . . .

WHAT YOU'LL LEARN IN THIS BOOK

In this book I'll teach you my simple Go with Your Gut Weight Loss Formula: a revolutionary approach to losing weight, healing your gut and loving your body and your life. You'll drop kilos and the mental chatter that weighs on your heart, keeps you feeling stuck and makes you feel less than fabulous in your body.

You'll learn to listen to that little intuitive voice inside that knows exactly what you need to eat, how you need to move and how you need to live your life – even if you suspect you've been ignoring it.

You'll get all the information and inspiration you need to lose weight and get your digestion going, but you'll also feel motivated to brighten up your career, relationships and spirituality – because all areas of your life are connected.

Best of all, you'll find a sense of ease. There will be less of the distracting 'should I, shouldn't I' drama in your head. You will feel grounded, supported and clear on what choices are best for your body and for your life. You will be thin from within.

Ready to get started?
Let's do this.

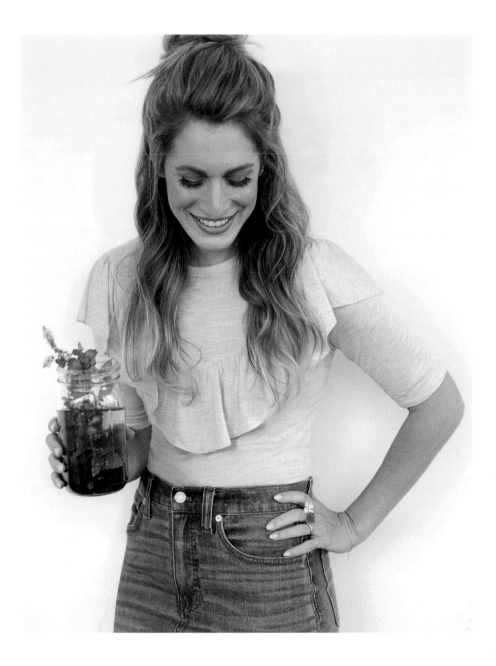

chapter one

CONFESSIONS
OF A
SERIAL DIETER

So many women I talk to are dealing with most (or all) of these symptoms:

♦ The inability to lose weight and keep it off

♦ Uncomfortable bloating and puffiness

♦ Constipation and/or diarrhoea

♦ Feeling tired, even after eight hours of sleep

♦ Dull skin and/or embarrassing acne

♦ Stress and anxiety that never seem to go away

♦ Trouble falling or staying asleep

And a lot of these women are drinking green juice and going to Pilates at the weekends.

If you picked up this book, you have weight-loss goals, but it's likely you are experiencing some of these other symptoms, too. At this point, I'm sure you're frustrated with two-week cleanses and strict meal plans because they don't fit into your life over the long term.

I'M JUST LIKE YOU

It can be easy (and wonderful) to lose weight and feel incredible in your body, but I didn't always know that. A few years ago, I had so many weight-loss and lifestyle tools swimming around in my head that I felt like I didn't know where to start.

I tried everything – the 3-Day Diet, the Cabbage Soup Diet, Weight Watchers, the 21 Day Fix and more – to muscle my body into a weight I deemed was acceptable for my height and frame. I tried to exist on minimal calories to 'get back on track' after holidays. I bought supplements that promised to boost my metabolism and help me shed weight effortlessly. I was looking for everything outside of me to 'fix' me.

MY HISTORY OF DIETING

When I was growing up, my mum cooked nourishing, real food 90 per cent of the time, so I developed a deep love of food and eating. I mean, who wouldn't, when served gourmet dishes like coq au vin and lemon meringue pie on a regular basis? The problem started when I began picking up messages from TV shows and commercials, in magazines and from the other girls at school that I needed to be on someone else's plan to be happy. So I'd stick to wholemeal-bread sandwiches, carrot or celery sticks and anything 100 calories or less in a tiny package. By the end of the day, I would be famished and so would ferret around in the kitchen cupboards looking for cookies, crisps and anything chewy and sweet I could lay my hands on.

The first real diet I remember going on was the 3-Day Diet, a low-calorie plan of hot-dogs and cottage cheese that's supposed to trigger quick weight loss. My mum would do it every other month or so to slim down, and one month I decided to join her. I think I lost one kilo, which I immediately gained back when I returned to my 'normal' way of eating.

My obsession with losing weight and wanting to feel great in my body continued into my twenties, as I tried to find myself and figure out what course my life was taking.

I was always trying to eat the most food for the least amount of calories. I loved eating, just like my dad, and I never wanted to feel deprived or like I was eating tiny portions. I would load up on low-fat versions of popcorn and crisps – the sort of stuff you can eat by the bowlful for about fifty calories. The problem was I never felt physically satiated because there's not much real nutrition in those foods.

I didn't understand how to properly feed myself because I was so disconnected from my body.

WHAT SHIFTED THINGS FOR ME

You might be thinking, 'Okay, so how did you do it, Robyn? How did you finally lose weight and turn your story into your life's work without it all feeling so hard?'

Well, it starts with a love story. It may sound like I'm about to share a story of falling in love with a person, but it's even deeper, bigger and better than that. It was about falling in love with my life. It did start with a special person, though . . .

When my husband, Scott, and I first started dating, shopping at the farmers' market and cooking was a way for us to connect. I dropped the packaged food and picked up the best of the best. I noticed that the more 'real' foods I ate, the less I craved commercialised fruit snacks and the less I was turning to food for comfort.

I was starting to feel better in my body, but it wasn't just about eating healthier food, it was also about the time I spent in the kitchen. While I was cooking, I wasn't trying to 'fix' anything. I felt creative and inspired. Cooking was my first meditation practice. It was a way for me to slow down and be in the moment. This newfound sense of being present was revolutionary for me.

Cooking was not only the first step in my body and diet transformation, it was the catalyst for a new career that lit me up.

Once I got cooking, I couldn't stop talking about the yummy foods I was creating on a regular basis. My friends could tell how passionate I was becoming about food and nutrition and one of them suggested that I check out the Institute for Integrative Nutrition (IIN), the world's largest health coach–training programme. One week later, I enrolled.

I was terrified of taking such a big leap, but every fibre in my body, my gut, was telling me to go for it.

> I WAS STILL OVEREATING AND OVER-SNACKING AT NIGHT. HEALTHY HAD ALMOST BECOME ANOTHER DIET FOR ME, AND IT STILL FELT LIKE MY BODY WAS SOMETHING I WAS TRYING TO FIX.

Shortly after graduating from IIN, I built a successful coaching practice on how to fit healthy eating and cooking into busy lives. I had finally found my path. I was doing something that I was excited about, and a layer of what I refer to as 'emotional weight' was being shed.

I was definitely healthier, but still struggling with my physical weight. I felt I was five to seven kilos heavier than I knew my body wanted to be; my outsides weren't matching my insides.

HOW I MOVED TO THE NEXT LEVEL

My biggest body, weight and mind shift happened when I focussed on nourishing my gut and taking care of myself, from the inside out. When my husband and I began talking about starting a family, I shifted my focus from 'How skinny can I be?' to 'How can I create the most ideal 'home' for my future baby to live in?' And then it dawned on me: our bodies are our homes. So shouldn't we treat them right?

I let go of trying to look a certain way. I slowed down even more at meal times and chewed my food completely. I began to focus on the foods (and the activities) that made me feel my best. And guess what? The foods that made me feel (and eventually look) my best were those deeply nourishing foods, the foods that feed and balance the microbiome (aka your gut).

WHY THE GUT?

Your gut is the centre of your being – it digests and assimilates nutrients from the food that you eat. It's where the majority of your immune system resides, and it also plays an important role in mood and hormones. If I wanted to build the best home possible, it made sense that my gut was the place to start. The more I dived into the gut-health world, the more I saw that healing the gut would resolve so many of my clients' issues (even the most stubborn ones). By focussing on healing the gut, these women were able to calm their digestive issues and also calm their out-of-control emotional eating.

As I mentioned at the beginning of this book, there are three main reasons why gut health is directly linked to reaching your ideal weight:

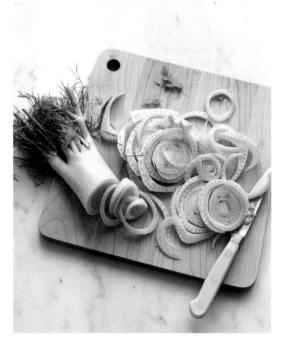

 1 *A healthy gut better absorbs nutrients from the food you are eating*

 2 *A healthy gut knows exactly what you need to feel your best*

 3 *A healthy gut means a happier you*

1. A HEALTHY GUT BETTER ABSORBS NUTRIENTS FROM THE FOOD YOU ARE EATING

Contrary to much diet advice out there, it's not just what you eat or the number of calories you consume but how your body is using those calories that counts. The digestive system's main jobs are to break down the food you eat and to absorb and assimilate the nutrients from that food.

You might be eating nutritious, whole foods most of the time but still feel foggy, uninspired and generally less than your brightest self. Why? Because if your gut isn't in tip-top shape, it's not properly absorbing all the vitamins and nutrients from your food, which means your cells don't have the fuel they need to do their jobs. It's like having a jewellery box full of diamonds but not having the key to unlock the box to wear those beautiful gems!

Your body may also enter starvation mode, known in scientific circles as metabolic adaptation, where it conserves and stores energy by holding on to fat. This also happens on low-calorie plans. If your body isn't getting enough nutrients, the brain's hypothalamus and pituitary glands work with other endocrine glands to retain calories (i.e. conserve resources) so that your body systems keep functioning.

When your digestion is functioning optimally, your gut absorbs the nutrients it needs from the healthy food you are eating and then signals to your brain that you are satisfied. You won't enter starvation mode because you aren't starving for nutrients. Your body won't need to store excess fat for energy because it trusts that it will get the nutrients it needs when it needs them.

With a healthy gut, you naturally eat a little less (because you are getting more out of what you are eating), dropping those stubborn extra kilos while maintaining optimal energy levels.

YOUR BODY WON'T NEED TO STORE EXCESS FAT FOR ENERGY BECAUSE IT TRUSTS THAT IT WILL GET THE NUTRIENTS IT NEEDS WHEN IT NEEDS THEM.

2. A HEALTHY GUT KNOWS EXACTLY WHAT YOU NEED TO FEEL YOUR BEST

Most weight-loss plans don't work because we ignore our bodies in favour of the latest trend. When our gut instinct pops up and says, 'Hell no', we ignore it because a louder voice is telling us these stories:

- My best friend Jess lost five kilos doing Whole30 so I should start that plan this week.
- All the wellness girls on Instagram are eating tons of organic almond butter, raw chocolate and ten bananas a day – I guess that means I can, too!
- Such-and-such a celebrity drinks a shot of apple cider vinegar before each meal. I'm on it!

When you learn to listen to your body, it will lead you to exactly the foods, workouts and life choices that are best for you at each moment. This isn't something a diet will accomplish for you. You must go deeper and connect to your intuition.

What I found to be the key missing piece during my years of dieting – and the reason I couldn't lose weight for most of my life – was self-trust. I didn't trust my body one bit. When I craved and ate pizza, I suffered from self-judgment and felt gross. When I ate salad, I would at first feel good for making the 'right choice,' but shortly afterwards would feel hungry and would then often end up snacking into oblivion, cancelling out any benefits from eating the salad.

I didn't trust my gut and the signals it was giving me. I wasn't listening.

After years of berating my thighs for not being thin enough and constantly comparing myself to other (smaller, better, more successful, blah blah) women, I'm now relieved to be at peace with my body and life, and I want you to feel that way too.

Our bodies are designed to seek optimum health. Your body is on your side and wants you to feel good. When you give it a chance, it will tell you exactly what it needs. This is the more spiritual side of gut health – it's about reconnecting with your intuition and reconditioning yourself to trust it.

 ## 3 A HEALTHY GUT MEANS A HAPPIER YOU

Many experts refer to the gut as your 'second brain' because it contains millions of neurons, which are quite sensitive to emotion. Multiple scientific studies have proven that our brain and gut are connected by an extensive network of neurons, chemicals and hormones that constantly provide feedback about how hungry we are and about whether or not we're experiencing stress, sadness or even anger. These emotions can trigger a reaction in your gut.

Have you ever felt your belly flip after receiving an e-mail you were dreading? That's the brain–gut connection in action. This is meant to work in our favour: just thinking of what you are going to eat for lunch can release digestive juices and prepare your body to eat before you even take your first bite.

The brain–gut connection is a two-way street, however: tummy troubles can impact your mood and happiness. Do you know what serotonin is? It's your body's 'feel good' neurotransmitter, which means it carries signals along and between your nerves. Serotonin is responsible for regulating a number of body processes, such as sleep and digestion, but its main role is to regulate anxiety, happiness and mood. In fact, low levels of serotonin have been associated with depression. It's estimated that 90 per cent of your serotonin is made in your digestive tract, and that the production of this chemical is reliant on healthy gut bacteria.

If your gut is a mess from poor food choices, stress and other factors, you're never going to feel the way you imagine your 'goal weight' to feel. In other words, even if you reach your goal weight on the scales, without a healthy gut, you may still feel bloated, unsettled and uncomfortable in your body. If you have a history of dieting (and self-doubt) like me, there's a good chance your gut bacteria is way off, and this is what's stopping you from feeling and looking the way you want to.

WHAT IS THE MICROBIOME AND WHY IS IT IMPORTANT?

The microbiome is all the tiny microbes that live in and on our bodies. These little bugs mainly help with digestion and fighting infection, but they also play a role in our moods and determining our level of happiness.

Your microbiome begins to develop at birth. Babies get covered in microbes as they pass through the birth canal and receive more via their mother's milk. The microbiome continues to grow and change as a result of familial, dietary and environmental factors.

So, what does the microbiome do? All these little guys help to extract vitamins and other nutrients from the foods you eat and deliver it to all your cells. You can think about your microbiome each time you eat kale and quinoa, as it helps get all the goodness out of these foods and into your body. It's also an essential component to immune function. Seventy to 80 per cent of your immune tissues are located within your digestive system. The gut is often the first entry point for pathogens, so keeping it healthy is what helps you avoid illness.

THIS GOES DEEP

When I finally focussed on nourishing my gut with both the foods and the mindful eating practices I teach in this book, my physical body started to look the way I had always imagined it in my mind. I lost those stubborn five kilos, but, more importantly, I got off the diet rollercoaster and finally felt at home in my body.

Yes, this is deep, and yes, this whole gut health–weight loss connection is more complicated than just taking a probiotic pill and munching on some greens. Don't worry, though: I'm going to give you a formula for your new way of eating and living, and a manageable plan that you can put in place tomorrow, or even today. But first, we need to get clear on where you are starting from and what your specific goals are. In the next chapter, I'll walk you through just that.

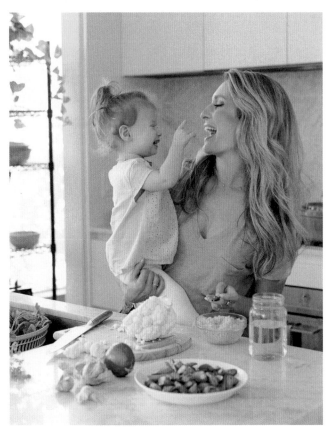

START
WHERE
YOU ARE

◇

YOU DESERVE TO FEEL
AMAZING IN YOUR BODY —
INSIDE AND OUT. YOU CAN BE
A SPIRITUAL PERSON AND STILL
WANT TO LOSE WEIGHT.

If you're hesitant to say you wish your dress size were smaller, you can let out a sigh of relief because here's the truth: you can love and appreciate your body as it is right now and still want to lose weight. Your body is your business, and if you want to look and/or feel different and that desire comes from you – not from the media, your mum or your boyfriend – it's all right to take action to make your dream body your real body.

Your body and your soul work in tandem, and the better you take care of your physical body, the more able you are to take care of your spirit.

Yes, there are a lot of things that are more important than how much you weigh. In fact, almost everything is more important than how much you weigh.

Now that we've got that out of the way, let's get to work! In this moment, how good do you feel in your body on a scale of one to ten? If that number is less than a nine or ten, you're in the right place. Make a mental note of your number as a way to get honest with yourself and start making loving, gradual changes from this point on so you can feel happy in your body, calm around food, and inspired in your life.

Whenever I get started with a new client, I always use the first session for us to get clear on where they currently are and where they want to be. If you don't know where you want to be, how will you know when you've got there?

@ *I created a special workbook to support the practices that I'm teaching you in this book. This will give you a place to get clear on your goals, track your progress and put what you're learning into real action. Head to robynyoukilis.com/books to download your free copy!*

A NOTE ON DIGESTIVE DISORDERS

The tips and recipes in this book will help virtually anyone improve their gut health, but there are a few more serious digestive disorders that require particular attention. I've summarised them below. If you think you may have one of these conditions, please talk to your doctor before undertaking any new plan or supplement regime.

Leaky gut, also known as intestinal permeability, occurs when particles are able to 'leak' from your intestine into your bloodstream. This causes inflammation throughout your body, leading to a variety of issues, such as food sensitivities, autoimmune diseases, malabsorption of nutrients, skin conditions (like acne and psoriasis) and mood issues.

Crohn's disease and ulcerative colitis are both major categories of inflammatory bowel disease (IBD). Crohn's disease is a chronic inflammatory condition of the gastrointestinal tract. Ulcerative colitis is a chronic inflammatory condition limited to the colon, otherwise known as the large intestine. Both Crohn's and ulcerative colitis have similar symptoms such as diarrhoea, urgent need to move bowels, abdominal cramps and pain, as well as the sensation of not being able to get it all out when you go to the toilet. General symptoms associated with IBD include loss of appetite, weight loss, fatigue, night sweats and loss of a normal menstrual cycle.

Small Intestinal bacterial overgrowth, commonly known as SIBO, is when there is excessive bacteria in the small intestine. When in proper balance, the bacteria in the colon help digest foods and assist the body in absorbing essential nutrients. However, when this bacteria invades and takes over the small intestine, it can lead to poor nutrient absorption and digestive discomfort, and may even lead to damage of the stomach lining. Symptoms include nausea, bloating, gas, diarrhoea, malnutrition, joint pain, fatigue, skin rashes, eczema, asthma and even depression. If you have SIBO, you probably need a diet very different from the one offered in this book, so I recommend sticking with the emotional teaching components and guidelines on 'how' to eat rather than focussing on the specific foods themselves.

Celiac disease, an autoimmune disease that can occur in genetically predisposed people, is an allergy to gluten that leads to damage in the intestines. When people with celiac disease eat gluten, their bodies mount an immune response that attacks the small intestine, specifically the villi, which are small fingerlike projections that line the small intestine and help with nutrient absorption. When the villi become damaged, nutrients cannot be properly absorbed into the bloodstream. The symptoms of celiac disease can vary greatly and are different in children and adults. The most common signs for adults are diarrhoea, fatigue and weight loss; other symptoms not directly related to the digestive system include anaemia, mouth ulcers, headaches and fatigue, joint pain, itchy skin, loss of bone density, and nervous system issues, such as problems with balance or numbness in the hands and feet.

DEFYING OLD STORIES

Being a wellness babe is not about being the same size you were when you were twenty-four. Getting stuck in that used-to-be mind-set will keep you feeling frustrated no matter how much progress you've actually made.

When my client Sandy came to me, she couldn't believe what she saw in the mirror. She had always been naturally skinny and was not used to seeing curves on her body. Sandy was so stuck on how she used to look that she felt crappy no matter how many positive shifts she made in her life (or kilos she lost).

Before we started working together, Sandy was lucky if she pooped once a week – and she thought this was normal. She had no idea what kale, kombucha or sauerkraut were and her family was not on board with her healthy lifestyle goals. Together we did the practical work, but we also did the inner, emotional work. We looked at the things that were weighing on Sandy, more than just a few extra kilos around her hips – what I refer to as 'emotional weight'.

Now she has a garden where she grows all sorts of vegetables (including kale!) and makes her own sauerkraut. Her sixteen-year-old daughter regularly asks for the recipes from my first book, *Go with Your Gut*, for dinner, and they go to the gym together once a week. She poops daily and has a lot of good gut tools at hand for when it feels like her life and body aren't flowing.

She's also much nicer to herself. She makes breakfast most days, she's investing in herself both personally and professionally and she speaks more kindly to herself. She's crafting her self-acceptance, while still continuing to move forwards with her body and life goals.

Does she still have days when she looks in the mirror and her thoughts start to drift to a negative place? Sure, but she's making progress every day and learning to trust herself more and more. Instead of focussing on how she used to be, she's envisioning, and blossoming into, a life that's brighter, more expansive and more beautiful than what's past.

YOUR PERSONAL GOALS

Pull out that pretty journal you've got, or just a notepad, and jot down three specific goals you have for yourself and your health. Weight loss can be one of them, but I encourage you to focus on other positive changes you want to see in your life, too. Feel free to flick back through the client stories I've shared so far for some inspiration.

GIVE YOURSELF A VISUAL

As we get started, I'm going to make one small request: take a photo of yourself right now at the beginning of this journey. Why a photo? As humans, we're wired to see our weak spots, the places where we're vulnerable or need improvement. This is why when you look in the mirror, all you see is what you wish were different, even if your best friend says you look amazing. I suggest taking photos because you can't always trust you'll see positive change in the moment. It's not to bash yourself with; it's just a check-in to see exactly where you are now. Notice how you look physically, but also energetically and emotionally.

You may want to take a moment with a journal and write down what's coming up for you. Then set a reminder on your calendar for one month and three months from the date of your initial photo. Use these photos to see how far you've come. Heads up: taking photos of yourself can bring up lots of emotions.

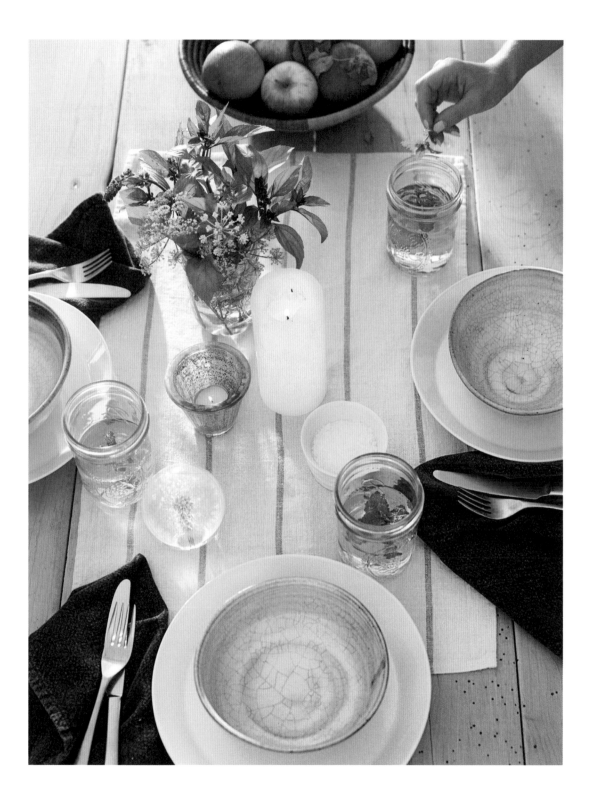

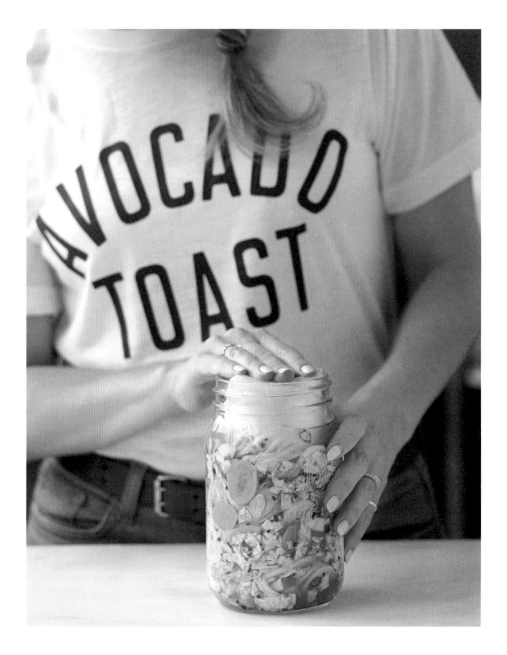

chapter two

THE GO WITH YOUR GUT FORMULA

THE GO WITH YOUR GUT WEIGHT LOSS FORMULA

The Go with Your Gut Weight Loss Formula is life-changing, especially if, like me, you're a recovering dieter. You may have picked up this book for the recipes, and even if you only make the recipes and do nothing else, you'll see a huge transformation in your body and life. Cooking changes everything, which is why this book is so recipe-focussed.

However, if you want to be like Amy, who lost three kilos and, more important, let go of her guilt around eating and food, keep reading. Spend some time with the next few chapters to upgrade everything you are doing in the kitchen.

My approach to weight loss is based on gut health and smart cooking as well as simple daily practices that shift your mindset and energy. GO WITH YOUR GUT is a four-part formula with the most important practices to incorporate into your everyday life. You can implement these practices whether you cook your meals at home, eat on the road, or somewhere in between. GO WITH YOUR GUT is a food and lifestyle framework to ultimately make your own.

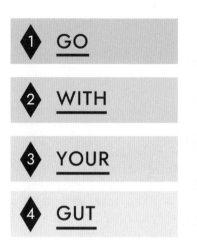

1. GO

2. WITH

3. YOUR

4. GUT

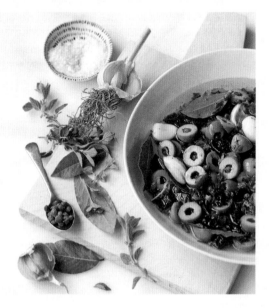

STEP ◆1

GO

We're going to get right into straight talking, because that's who I am and that's what's worked for hundreds of my clients. You need to be **GO**-ing first thing in the morning – and yes, I mean pooping.

You should have a nice smooth bowel movement – well-formed and easy to pass – first thing in the morning. I know it's not the nicest thing to talk about, but it's essential to the good-gut approach, and you and I both know how amazing a good poop feels. There's a reason for that: you're flushing toxins out of your body and preparing your tummy to digest your next meal.

So how can you make sure you're pooping every day? The first step is to drink a big glass of water as soon as you wake up. I keep an extra-large glass filled with filtered water on my bedside table and drink it down as soon as I open my eyes and sit up in the morning.

You can step it up by drinking warm or hot water with lemon, but the most important thing is that you're just getting water of some sort down the hatch, and a good amount of it – at least 350ml and as much as 750ml.

Ready to bump it up a notch further? Try my Go with Your Gut Shot first thing in the morning to get things moving: simply combine 30–50ml pure aloe vera juice, 1 tablespoon raw apple cider vinegar and a squeeze of lemon juice and shoot it down just like you'd take a shot of tequila with the girls on a Saturday night.

WATER, WATER EVERYWHERE!

Drinking plenty of quality water is essential for good health and weight loss. Here are a few of my top tips about your new favorite beverage du jour from my first book, Go with Your Gut:

◆ Don't drink water with meals: it will dilute your gastric juices. Aim to finish any beverages thirty minutes before each meal and wait an hour after each meal before drinking more.

◆ Avoid adding ice to your water – it puts out your belly's 'fire'. Your digestive system does better with room temperature or warm water.

◆ Make sure you are drinking enough water each day. Here is a good formula to calculate how much you need: divide your body weight in kilograms by thirty and this is the number of litres you should drink each day.

◆ I recommend investing in a home filtration system of some kind and drinking out of glass containers whenever possible (for my favorite water bottles and filters, head to robynyoukilis.com/books).

STEP 2

WITH

Simplify your food **WITH** the Good Gut Rule of Five. I created the Good Gut Rule of Five to show you exactly what to put on your plate at lunch and dinner.

Eating in this way will ensure that you are getting a balance of both macro- and micronutrients, as well as my favourite gut healing superfoods.

Aim to include one ingredient from each of the five categories opposite for a complete and balanced meal.

MACRO- AND MICRONUTRIENTS

Macronutrients are the calorific components of our foods that most of us are familiar with: carbohydrates, fats and proteins. Micronutrients are the vitamins, minerals, trace elements, phytochemicals and antioxidants within our foods that are essential for proper cellular function and good health. Many processed and packaged foods contain plenty of calories, but are lacking in micronutrients (which is why you can seem to eat and eat and eat these foods without being really 'full'). I created the Good Gut Rule of Five as an easy way to ensure you're getting a healthy balance of both macro- and micronutrients in the majority of your meals.

 GREENS

Kale, spring greens, rocket, spinach, lettuce . . . I love them all. Aim to have at least two or three big handfuls of greens with most meals. Greens do it all when it comes to gut health and weight loss: they're packed with fibre, which helps fill you up and keep you regular. Plus, leafy green veggies are some of the most nutrient-dense foods, and when you are filling your cells with nutrients (I mean real nutrition, not just calories!), you have more energy and fewer cravings.

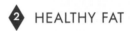 HEALTHY FAT

Avocado, olive and flax oils, almonds, butter from grass-fed cows (so the cows have healthy guts too!) and coconut oil all count here. Add 1–2 tablespoons of oil, 25–50g of nuts or ¼–½ of an avocado at each meal for a good dose of flavour and satiation. Plus, fats are essential for proper absorption of most vitamins and minerals. I used to be terrified of fats but now I include them as part of every meal and am lighter than I've ever been.

◆3 PROTEIN

Wild salmon, grass-fed beef, organic chicken, tempeh, sprouted lentils and tinned wild sardines are some examples of great go-to protein options on the Go with Your Gut Weight Loss Formula. Protein keeps you full and stabilises your blood sugar, so you won't keep dipping into your raw chocolate stash or crash halfway through your afternoon meetings.

◆4 FERMENTED FOOD

Including fermented foods on your plate is the good gut secret to weight loss through a healthy microbiome (you need all that great bacteria throughout the day to keep your digestion humming!). Examples include raw sauerkraut, fermented beetroot, fermented carrots or radishes and kimchi. Try adding 1–3 tablespoons at each meal and feel free to work your way up to 75g or more. If you're not used to the taste of fermented veggies, you can try mixing them with avocado to mellow the flavour. Ideally, you should have a fermented veggie with your meal, but if not, you can get your daily dose of probiotics from kombucha, kefir, yogurt, or any of the other sweeter fermented foods.

◆5 COOKED VEGETABLES

Having a cooked veggie or two with my meal (in addition to greens) always makes the meal feel more filling. Roasted courgettes, broccoli, sweet potatoes, squash and carrots are all delicious examples, but this can really be any vegetables. I try to roast a bunch of anything that's in season at least once or twice a week so I always have some cooked veggies on hand and ready to go. If you're on the run, many takeaway spots and fancy restaurants have great options these days.

Keep your meals simple and nourishing with these five components.

 Whether you're making a recipe from this book, or simply compiling a plate from your local salad bar, I want to see your Good Gut Rule of Five meals! Snap a photo and post to Instagram, Facebook, or Twitter – make sure to tag #gowithyourgutdiet and @RobynYoukilis so I can see your delicious photos and be inspired!

WHAT ABOUT BREAKFAST?

The recipes in this book will cover you for breakfast; whether you're having a Power Parfait, a gut-friendly smoothie or a savoury option, you'll likely be hitting on many of the Rule of Five categories without even thinking about it! I've found that this rule is most applicable (and most helpful) for the other meals of the day, where we tend to get more confused as to what exactly belongs on our plate.

STEP ◆3

YOUR

Take **YOUR** time for you before everyone else in the space between your day and your evening. This is where things get messy for most of us, even after eating a solid lunch and maybe even making it to that after-work spin class.

Take a moment to refocus on your body, yourself, your needs and your goals in the transition. Whether you're heading back to your quiet studio flat, or going home to your kids and husband and dog (who all need you, all at once), take a few

tip

Are you a stay-at-home mum or an at-home anything? You can practise this, too. Go for a walk, lock yourself in a quiet room, lay down on the ground – do something to mark the transition from work to home (even if the physical transition doesn't exist).

minutes to check in with yourself and transition from work life to your home life, whatever that means for you. This step is key in breaking up with mindless eating habits and dropping the emotional weight.

If your home space allows you to have a few calm minutes for you, you can do this as soon as you get home. If everything is in your face all at once as soon as you walk in the door, you might need to sit in your car or find a park bench where you can have a few minutes. Put your phone down – you can check it later. This is your moment to check in with your body and brain and recalibrate. Take a few deep breaths, drop your shoulders and make yourself a cup of tea or drink a big glass of water if you can. Come back into yourself – acknowledge what happened during your day and then set an intention for the evening. Are you going to cook yourself dinner? Do some light yoga? Call your mum? What do you want your evening to look (and feel) like?

This moment of recalibration is what sets you up for real and sustainable weight loss success – it's essential in closing the gap between how you want to spend your evening and the post-work autopilot that so many of us find ourselves in.

STEP ◆4
GUT

Finally, and probably most important, nourish your **GUT**. You want to be adding extra key nutrients and supplements to love your gut up. Yes, you want to be eating the food from this book first and foremost, but you'll probably need to start taking some probiotics (or remember to take them) and adding in a little extra fibre, too.

One important tip about probiotics – I recommend taking them at night. This is when your digestive system is in its most relaxed state and your body can assimilate them best. Your organs, digestive system included, rest and repair while you're sleeping. Give your body time to digest your food at night by having an earlier dinner (ideally three to fours hours before bedtime) so you have space to process your food and the events of your day before you go to sleep.

The last piece of the Go with Your Gut Weight Loss Formula, and one of my own personal weight loss secret weapons, are my Good-Gut Jellies (page 165). Add these as a little treat after dinner to take in extra fibre, which is key for a good poop (which brings us full circle back to the first step of my Go with Your Gut Weight Loss Formula: make sure you GO!).

I'll talk more about probiotics and other key gut supplements on page 58.

The rest of the book builds on the Go with Your Gut Weight Loss Formula. We're starting with 'go' – that is, your morning routine – in the next chapter. So let's go!

WHAT ARE PRO- AND PREBIOTICS ANYWAY?

Probiotics are the good bacteria your gut needs to carry out digestion properly. Probiotics are found naturally in fermented foods like sauerkraut, kimchi, yogurt, miso, tempeh and more. The two primary organisms or strains of bacteria in probiotics are *Lactobacillus* and *Bifidobacterium*. We need both to properly break down and absorb our food so we can keep our metabolism humming fast and lose (or maintain) weight.

Prebiotics are nondigestible fibres that promote the growth of beneficial microorganisms in your intestines. Examples include apples, garlic, jicama, dandelion greens and onions. Think of them as a natural fertiliser that feeds your internal garden.

If you've had tummy troubles for years, the solution isn't to throw as many probiotics and prebiotics at it as you can. They might make you feel worse or keep you stuck on the toilet for days. Do your research, or work one-on-one with someone who can help you safely integrate these nutrients into your diet.

A note about antibiotics: antibiotics kill off bacteria – the bad and the good – so they can cause damage to your gut. If you absolutely must take them, be sure to take a probiotic supplement and eat plenty of probiotic-rich foods during your course of antibiotics to help restore the good bacteria in your gut.

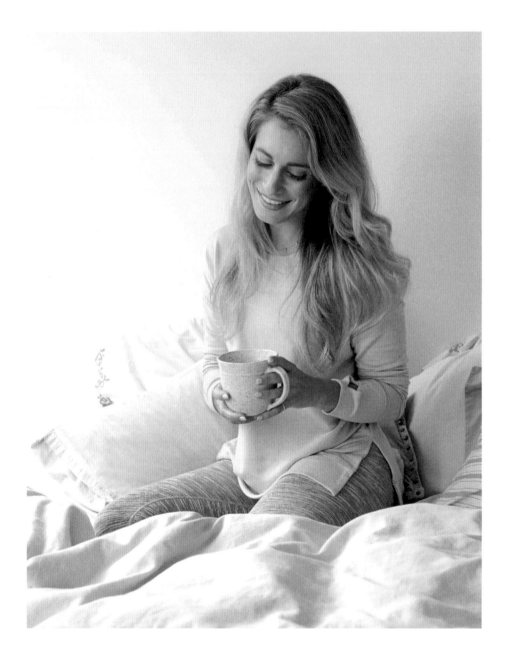

chapter three

YOUR
MORNING
ROUTINE

A s I sat up in my bed and took a little stretch, the sunshine beamed in on my face and I could hear the birds chirping outside my window. I thought to myself, 'Hello, beautiful day!' I made my way over to my meditation cushion and settled in for my Zen morning routine.

And then I woke up.

In reality, my morning actually looks more like this: my beautiful daughter is hungry and needs to be changed and fed immediately. My husband – the same. Just kidding! But he does have questions about our dinner plans that night, and my phone is pinging with email after email.

Morning 'routine'? Most days, it's a challenge just to find a moment to poop in peace!

WHY YOU MIGHT NOT BE GOING FOR NUMBER 2

Maybe you have your own version of my morning reality. I find the reason most of us are not going is because we aren't giving ourselves a moment to come into self at the beginning of the day. All the foods and recipes in this book will help you have nice, easy poops on the regular, but you also need to give your body the time and space to actually go.

When you anchor yourself in your body for a few minutes each morning, not only do you set yourself up for a good poop, you also set the tone for the rest of your day. You are in the driver's seat of your life. Once you are present in your body, you are more likely to make positive choices all day.

If you're like me and have a young child – or you're facing other circumstances that leave you rolling your eyes at the very thought of a morning routine – be reassured: you don't need to spend hours journalling or chanting on your yoga mat to reap the benefits of a little morning time.

MY MORNING MINUTE

Here's what I do most days: when I wake up, I place one hand on my heart and one hand on my belly and I take a few deep breaths. I say some version of the following to myself (think *Goodnight Moon*, but the morning self-care version) . . .

'Hi, I'm awake. How lovely is that? Good morning, body; good morning heart. I've got you. I'm here; this is me. These are my arms, this is my skin, this is my chest, this is my face. I've got you.'

When I take that moment to check in with myself, to start the day with ease and calm, not only am I more likely to feel grounded and happy, I'm also much more likely to make positive choices throughout my day.

This minute of calm is what I call my Morning Minute. It's a moment for me to connect with my mind and my body, to get my feet under me before the day gets ahead of me.

There's no one 'right' way to do your Morning Minute. Try out a few of the ideas below to figure out what feels best for you.

Yours may be:

♦ One minute of breathing deeply into your belly

♦ Listening to a short guided meditation

♦ Shaking your body out to your favourite song

♦ Writing in a journal

♦ Reading a snippet from an inspirational book

♦ Sipping a cup of tea alone

♦ Gently tapping on your body (or any light movement) to increase blood flow

Why is it so important to take this time to chill out? Science shows that mindfulness and meditation lead to decreased levels of stress hormones, like cortisol. One study in particular from Georgetown University's Medical Center showed that an eight-week course of daily mindfulness classes lowered inflammatory molecules and stress hormones by around 15 per cent. When stress hormones are high, they send messages to your body to store calories as fat, making it harder to lose weight – even if you're eating all the healthy stuff. No joke! High levels of stress hormones can also cause inflammation and other health issues that can keep you from feeling your best.

In addition, you cannot properly digest and absorb the nutrients from your food if you're stressed. Your nervous system exists in one of two states: the sympathetic nervous system (the fight-or-flight response that accompanies stress) or the parasympathetic nervous system. Your body is designed to primarily exist in the parasympathetic state, which controls homeostasis, your body's sense of balance and its ability to carry out digestion.

If your sympathetic nervous system is engaged too often, your digestion is impaired because the body is designed to use energy first for survival – it doesn't know the difference between your reaction to an angry e-mail from your boss and you jumping out of the way of a bad driver. If you're stressed, your body puts up the same defences and dedicates all energy to staying alive, leaving secondary processes like digestion weakened.

When you use your breathing, and take mini breaks, like my Morning Minute, to de-stress and get your body into the parasympathetic state, your digestive system can do its job. And as a bonus, you're also more likely to make decisions from a calm and clear place.

HOW TO PRACTICE DEEP-BELLY BREATHING

Deep-belly breathing is an easy and effective tool for weight loss and improved digestion. And yes, one minute of deep breathing really can change the course of your day.

♦ Start by setting a timer for one minute
♦ Put one hand on your chest and the other on your belly
♦ Now breathe deeply into your stomach, letting it get as big as possible on the inhale, then relax on the exhale
♦ Repeat continuously, inhaling and exhaling in this manner, until the timer goes off

It's really important to let your belly expand fully. We spend so much of our day sucking it in, and that suppresses digestion.

MISSED YOUR MORNING MINUTE?

Ideally you take your Morning Minute at the very start of the day. before it's time to be a mum, a busy executive, a student, (insert all the other hats you might wear daily). But if you missed it you have the power to hit reset and connect with how you want to feel in any moment. Even one minute can make all the difference.

Here are six practical ways you can hit refresh on your day:

1 On your next visit to the toilet, add in one minute of deep-belly breathing

2 Go to lunch with a co-worker and practise the art of listening

3 Call a friend just to say 'How are you?'

4 Go for a quick walk around the block on your lunch break . . . and leave your phone at your desk

5 Listen to a song that soothes you or moves you. Bonus points for dancing along

6 Write down five things you're grateful for

You can sprinkle these little check-ins throughout your day to feel more calm, focussed and at peace with what is. When you're in that state, you'll feel ready to tackle your big goals while appreciating exactly where you are today.

MAKE IT HAPPEN

What do you need to do to make sure this practice happens? Do you need to download a meditation app, set an alarm for fifteen minutes earlier than usual or tell your partner about your new routine?

Write down how you'll make it happen below. Consider anything else that needs to shift that you'll want to plan or prepare for.

Find additional inspiration or share your Morning Minute using #gowithyourgutdiet

BREAKFAST IS SERVED

This first meal of the day can be a meditative check-in in and of itself, and feel just as awesome as your Morning Minute. Breakfast is an important part of my approach because in all my years of coaching I've found that my clients are so much less likely to binge later in the day if they've had a balanced breakfast (i.e. something more than a green juice or bagel with coffee). This is because when we deprive our bodies of nutrients, they overcompensate when we finally do feed them.

Despite the fact that we know we should eat breakfast, many women still struggle with this meal, or skip it because they just can't deal with it.

For years, I loved the time I spent in the morning making myself breakfast (remember what I said about cooking being my first meditation? It still is a grounding practice for me). I loved making beautiful, Instagram-worthy plates such as perfect scrambled eggs piled high with spicy arugula, fermented hot sauce, and sourdough toast. I was fortunate to have a job and a life that allowed, and actually encouraged, me to take this time each day.

I love this meal now, but everything changed when I got pregnant, and then again when I had my daughter, Navy.

During pregnancy, I couldn't even stomach the thought of eggs or greens. And spending any time over the hob? No thank you.

My cravings changed, my body changed, my life changed. And so my breakfast had to change, too.

I needed a new breakfast – something that would fuel my morning, that I loved eating and that I could make ahead of time or quickly on the spot when I didn't have time to prepare anything. After much experimentation, the Power Parfait was born (see pages 36–7). It's basically an upgraded yogurt, fruit and granola bowl, and was the recipe that triggered my easy post-baby weight loss.

Why? Because I listened to what my gut needed. Instead of trying to force myself to eat something that I thought was the 'healthiest' option based on what I had read (and even loved), I listened to my body and what it needed – something I'll be teaching you how to do for yourself in the chapters to come.

The other important factor of this breakfast was that it created a consistent routine in my days when, as a new mum, my mornings were anything but consistent.

I created this recipe for me, but I quickly became aware of how it solved the breakfast conundrum for many of my clients, because it meets the following criteria:

♦ You can prepare a load of Power Parfaits at the same time and set yourself up for the week.

♦ But you don't have to do anything in advance – this breakfast can just as easily come together on the spot.

♦ It contains gut-friendly fibre, probiotics and prebiotics.

♦ It's packed with protein, which will keep you full for hours.

♦ It's absolutely delicious!

♦ And as a bonus: your little ones will probably love it, too.

One client wrote to me to say, 'I've been making yogurt parfaits on Sunday night. This has made the difference between my eating a healthy breakfast and grabbing something fast like a sugary muffin, or worse, skipping it.'

note

The Power Parfait, like a smoothie, is a perfect vehicle for superfoods (see page 59). You don't have to miss out on the fun superfood craze just because you don't have a super-duper blender!

This breakfast has the power to set your mornings free, whether you're a new mum or just in need of an easy, gut-friendly meal to start your day.

The following recipe makes one serving – if you're making enough to last you for the week, simply line up your containers and measure the ingredients into each one. Feel free to vary the fruit you use.

◇

POWER
PARFAIT
BLUEPRINT

Here's the basic formula I use when making my Power Parfait bowls. Each day is a little different because I like to switch up the fruit and granola, but the formula remains the same. For more fun variations and how you can mix up your parfaits, head to pages 82–83.

180g natural yogurt

20g plain oats

1 teaspoon chia seeds

2 tablespoons of protein powder

  (check out my faves at robynyoukilis.com/ books!)

Splash or two of homemade nut milk or water

75g fresh berries or other chopped fruit

30g low-sugar granola

1 Mix the first five ingredients together.

2 Top with the fruit and granola. Eat immediately or store in the fridge for later!

yogurt

Goat's milk is my favorite, but you can also use organic cow's milk, sheep's milk, or plain coconut milk or nut-based yogurt.

oats

Oats are rich in prebiotic fiber and make this bowl so much more satisfying than your average yogurt cup. You can skip this add-in if you're paleo or grain-free.

chia

Chia seeds are rich in fiber and help clean out your digestive tract. Chia seeds are also full of omega-3 fatty acids, which help fight internal inflammation and fuel your brain to produce more feel-good hormones like serotonin.

tip

GRAIN-FREE? USE A COMBINATION OF UNSWEETENED SHREDDED COCONUT AND SLIVERED ALMONDS IN PLACE OF THE OATS AND GRANOLA (OR USE A GRAIN-FREE GRANOLA).

If you're looking for one place to start on your gut health and weight loss journey, start with your morning.

Your breakfast and morning routine set the tone for the rest of the day. This could be the difference between feeling good about your body and great about your life, or feeling like nothing is working out. It's always worth the one extra minute of breathing, or those 10 extra minutes of breakfast prep on the weekend. When my mornings start the way I want them to, I feel like I'm riding with the rest of my day, instead of being pulled along.

note

If your gut is saying HELL NO . . . and you instinctively know that yogurt or a cold and sweet breakfast is not for you, go with your gut, my friend! If you're not really sure what is best for you, experiment! There are plenty of other gut-friendly breakfasts in this book—head to page 75 for more delicious options.

@ *Do you love your Power Parfait as much as I do? Take a photo of your favorite variation and post it to social media— make sure to tag me @RobynYoukilis and #gowithyourgutdiet so I can see your beautiful creations!*

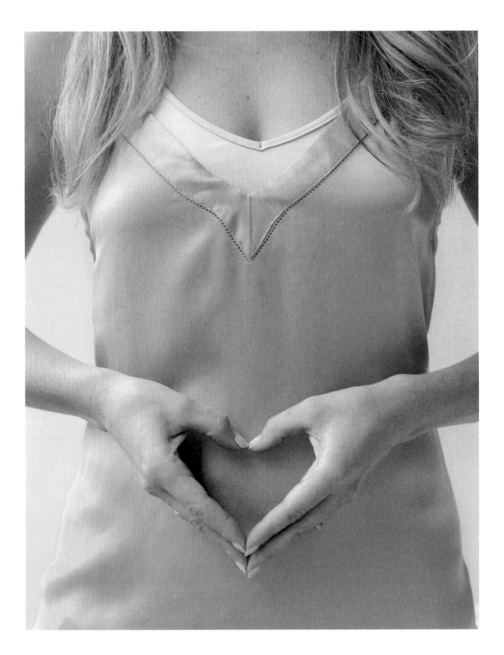

chapter four

THE 3-DAY GOOD GUT RESET

Let's recap what we've covered so far. We got crystal clear on your body image (on a scale of 1 to 10) and your current personal goals. I shared my Go with Your Gut Weight Loss Formula (which you can apply no matter what you have going on) and we did a morning makeover. Fun!

Now it's time to get into the program. In this chapter I'm sharing my 3-Day Good Gut Reset. It's a meal plan designed to jumpstart weight loss and give you a taste for how to structure your meals in a waist-friendly way, every day. Think of this as the starter program for you and your body to become familiar with new foods and methods of eating. To make life easy, I'm providing you with a shopping list and step-by-step instructions so all you have to do is shop and show up!

Can just three days of practice really make a difference? Yes it can! A study published by Scientific American indicates that changes to your diet can improve your gut bacteria within three or four days and it's possible to reset your hunger hormones in just three days. I'll dive into hunger hormones more in chapter five, but know for now that these chemical messengers can play a crucial role in the effectiveness of your weight loss efforts.

This 3-Day Reset does not look like a typical weight loss protocol, and I'll be totally honest: You will not lose 10 pounds in three days. This plan is designed to get you in a better place when it comes to your food choices and catalyze many more positive changes in your belly and life. Here's what my clients Jessica and Yvonne experienced:

> *Usually I give up easily on plans and protocols, but this one was different! I gave myself permission to make swaps when something didn't work for me. The end result? I lost 4 pounds of bloat!* — JESSICA

> *The thing I loved most about this reset was that it was so doable. I went into it focused on ease and peace, and it real was easy to follow along without the mental chatter I often find myself sorting through. I never felt hungry, I never felt deprived or like I was restricting. I felt like I was feeding myself well and felt taken care of.* — YVONNE

Here are some of the benefits you can expect to see (and feel) after completing this three-day plan:

- ◆ A calmer and flatter belly
- ◆ Less mindless snacking
- ◆ Feeling more confident in your meal prepping abilities
- ◆ And yes, you might lose some pounds

You'll notice a number of foods repeated or repurposed to minimise the total number of ingredients, allowing you to stop, drop and do this any day of the week. For this reason I purposely kept the meals simple and flexible. I also wanted to be a responsible coach and not make this feel diet-y or cleanse-y so that you don't jump into that mind-set of 'I'm starting my detox on Wednesday so until then I'll eat all the things.'

Just like the Power Parfait from chapter four, this is a template for you to follow, and eventually make your own.

Heads up – the first few days of any new routine can be the most challenging. Why? Because we live on autopilot and are used to eating what's easy and what's available (or what your partner/colleague/roommate is eating). You'll need to be a little bit more proactive and thoughtful when it comes to what you're putting in your body until this new way of eating becomes second nature.

If you're not ready to do this right now, that's okay! Feel free to scan it and come back at a time in your life that feels good to you. But if you know this is what you need, grab your grocery list and commit to it now.

SET YOUR INTENTION

My favourite part of a yoga class isn't laying down at the end of class in Savasana pose (although that's great, too) but when I'm asked by the teacher to set an intention for the class. I find this moment to pause so powerful – it immediately brings me into myself and is a sweet reminder of what any act of self-improvement is about. Yoga, as well as this reset, is not just about the physical benefits; it's about taking care of yourself at a deep level.

It's also helpful to have an intention to check back in with during more challenging moments. I recommend writing down your intention then reading it daily throughout your reset. If you're following along in your workbook, use the space provided there to clearly define your intentions.

Intention: *the thing that you plan to do or achieve: an aim or purpose*

Intentions don't have to be complicated or 'woo-woo'. They simply define the way you want to feel or what you want to focus on. I encourage you to focus on a feeling rather than on a specific physical goal. Here are some examples from people who have gone through this reset:

♦ My intention is to feel more confident in my daily food choices.
♦ I want to feel like I'm taking care of myself, instead of just reaching for what's available.
♦ I hope to feel more connected to my body and my intuition.

How many times have you sworn off sugar, bread or coffee on a Sunday night and by Tuesday morning found yourself grabbing a granola bar with a giant latte as you rush to the office?

Take a step back and ask yourself: how do I want to feel? What is the root of my desire to eat healthily? Brainstorm a few feelings that you are looking to introduce into your life. And then each time you have a choice to make (Side salad or fries? Happy hour or yoga? Another coffee or herbal tea?), make the one that aligns with that desired feeling.

Write for a few minutes to get all of your feeling- or word-focussed intentions out. You don't need to sum them up in a single or few words to start; just write everything down that comes to mind. After you've completed that part, go back and circle any words or feelings that jump out at you. Something that makes your heart sing or your belly feel calm would be great: intention words or feelings, for example.

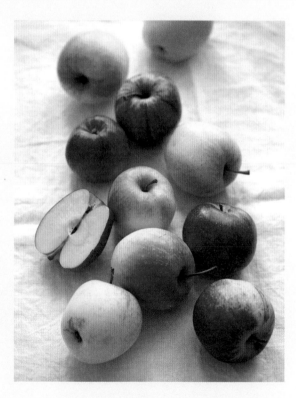

LET'S GO SHOPPING

Now that you've set your intention, it's time to go shopping! This list will be enough for one person for three days, plus some extra.

THE RESET: FRESH GROCERIES

- 1kg unsweetened natural yogurt of choice (goats', sheep's, organic cow's or plain coconut)
- 1 jar raw fermented sauerkraut
- Bone broth (at least 1 litre)
- 6 eggs
- Smoked salmon
- Rotisserie chicken
- 1 head green-leaf lettuce
- 500g carrots
- 1 avocado
- 1 bunch spring greens
- 2 bunches other leafy greens of choice (for soup: spinach, watercress, kale, mustards and/or more spring greens)
- Medium–large piece of fresh ginger
- 1 head garlic

- 1 yellow onion
- 1 bunch spring onions
- Raw Power Veggies of choice: fennel, jicama, celery and radishes (you can get one of each, or several of one)
- 1 head cauliflower
- 1 package stir-fry veggies (fresh or frozen)
- 2 or 3 small tubs of fresh berries (or 2 or 3 small apples)
- 2 or 3 lemons
- 2 bottles of kombucha (or homemade Fermented Fruit Soda, see page 181)
- Unfiltered quality apple juice (fresh and unpasteurised)
- Organic miso paste

THE BIG KOMBUCHA QUESTION

A lot of my clients ask me about the sugar in kombucha. Is it okay? The short answer is this: it depends. For 95 per cent of my clients, kombucha is key in supporting their health and helping them reduce their consumption of beverages like soda, coffee and alcohol. But yes, the sugar may be too much for some people. It all depends on your constitution and condition.

Most of the sugar in kombucha is what feeds the living, healthy bacteria. It gets broken down and the sugar is literally consumed by the culture. However, there's always a little residual sugar. Read the labels and pick a brand with the least amount of sugar, and drink no more than 125–175ml at a time.

The only way to know if kombucha and other fermented drinks work for you is to experiment. Try drinking a small glass every day for five days and take note of how it makes you feel. If you feel energised, clear headed and have no funny digestive stuff going on, stick with it! On the other hand, if you feel bloated, gassy or just plain tired when you drink kombucha regularly, it may not be right for you right now.

THE RESET: PANTRY STAPLES

You may already have these on hand – check before you start your 3-Day Good Gut Reset

- Protein powder of choice
- Chia seeds
- Psyllium husk
- Tinned wild salmon or sardines
- Nori sheets
- Plain, old-fashioned rolled oats
- Sea salt and black pepper
- Za'atar spice (or curry powder)

- Cayenne pepper
- Dijon mustard
- Tamari or coconut aminos
- Coconut oil or ghee
- Pumpkin seed oil (optional)
- Toasted sesame oil (optional)
- Teas (my favourite reset teas include nettle, dandelion and ginger)

GET YOUR RESET PREP ON

The next step is to do a little meal prep so you're not having to cook everything from scratch every time. Here's what I suggest doing the day before you start the Reset:

1 Make your Reset Power Parfaits
For your breakfast, grab three preserving jars, medium glasses or silicone containers. Into each container put 180g yogurt, 20g oats, 1 teaspoon chia seeds, 2 tablespoons protein powder and a splash of nut milk or water. Mix this all together and top with about 75g berries (or chopped apple) and a generous sprinkle of cinnamon. Put lids on your containers and pop them in the fridge.

ALTERNATIVE MAKE-AHEAD BREAKFASTS

Not everyone can digest the proteins in dairy. If you can't tolerate dairy, here are a few amazing breakfast alternatives that still fit the reset plan. Just make sure to update your shopping list accordingly.

♦ Blueberry Pie Smoothie (page 90)
♦ The Best Baked Porridge (page 77)
♦ Breakfast Salad (page 93)
♦ 2 hard-boiled eggs, ½ avocado, sauerkraut, drizzle of extra-virgin olive oil (bonus points if you can get some made-to-order steamed leafy greens on your plate, too!)

2 Roast your veggies
Preheat the oven to 220°C/gas mark 7. Wash the carrots and cauliflower and cut the carrots into sticks and the cauliflower into bite-sized florets. (Or, as a time-saving hack: buy prechopped veggies.) Place the carrots on one baking tray and the cauliflower on another. Toss the veggies with coconut oil and any chosen seasonings. Place the baking trays in the oven and cook until the carrots are tender and the cauliflower is browned. Set the cooked veggies aside (to fully assemble your meals in advance) or store in a sealed container in the fridge.

tip
Line your baking trays with greaseproof paper or aluminium foil for easy cleanup!

3 Wash and prep your greens
Wash your greens well (all of them) and then pat dry. You can also chop any leaf lettuce or kale at this point.

4 Make some Good-Gut Jellies
This is the easiest prep step of all: in a medium container, combine 350ml apple juice and 6 tablespoons psyllium husk. Mix well and divide evenly among three small containers. Place in the fridge to firm up. If you forget this step, no problem – you can make the jellies and let them set for a few minutes and they'll still be good to go.

5 Make some Healing Greens Soup
This soup takes only about 20 minutes to make, but if you're like me and want dinner done in five, you'll need to make it in advance. You can find the full recipe on page 112.

Extra credit
You can also prep your lunches in advance by filling three large lunch boxes with the ingredients for each meal listed in the plan that follows (see page 46).

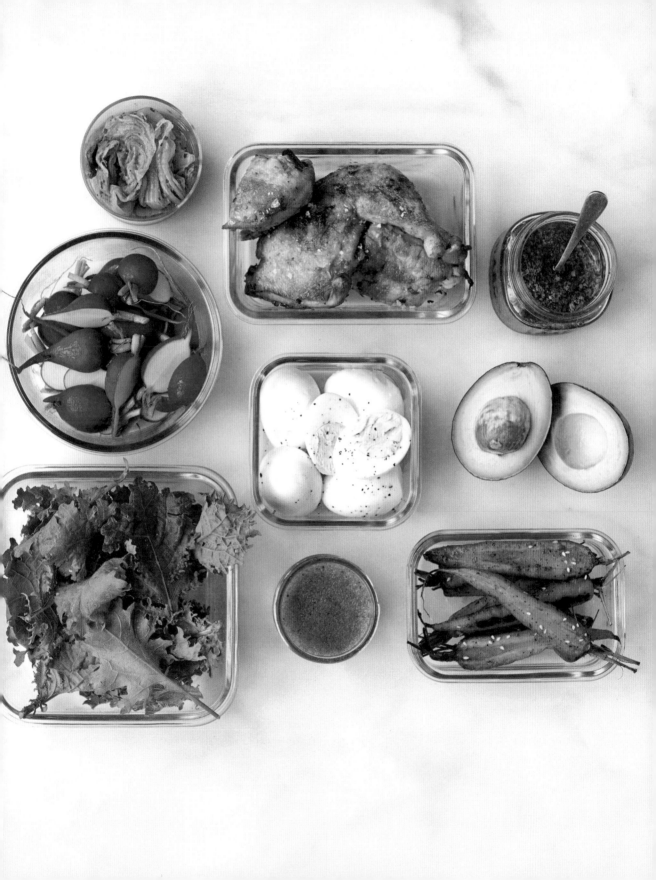

THE 3-DAY MEAL PLAN

DAY 1

AM: 115–175ml hot water with lemon and 700ml–1 litre plain water with a pinch of sea salt

Breakfast: Reset variation of Power Parfait (see page 44), tea or coffee with 1 teaspoon coconut oil or ghee mixed in

Optional Mid-morning Probiotic Pick-me-up: 125–175ml kombucha or Fermented Fruit Soda (page 181)

Lunch: A Good Gut Rule of Five Plate (see pages 26–7): green-leaf lettuce (as much as you like), about 100g roasted carrots, a small tin of wild salmon or sardines, ¼ avocado, and some sauerkraut. Dress with juice from the sauerkraut, a light drizzle of olive oil and a squeeze of lemon juice and season with salt and pepper. I also like to add a dollop of Dijon mustard for salmon and for dipping roasted veggies.

Snack: 240ml bone broth and about 150g roasted cauliflower

Dinner: Healing Greens Soup with an egg (cooked however you'd like) and a drizzle of sesame oil

After-Dinner Treat: A good-Gut Jelly and a mug of herbal tea

DAY 2

AM: 115–175ml hot water with lemon and 700ml–1 litre plain water with a pinch of sea salt

Breakfast: Reset variation of Power Parfait (see page 44), tea or coffee with 1 teaspoon coconut oil or ghee mixed in

Optional Mid-morning Probiotic Pick-me-up: 125–175ml kombucha or Fermented Fruit Soda (page 181)

Lunch: Spring Green Salad Wraps with smoked salmon or turkey and avocado (page 100)

Snack: Mug of Healing Greens Soup, sliced Raw Power Veggies (see page 42 – as much as you like)

Dinner: A Good Gut Rule of Five Plate: pile of steamed greens (as much as you like), 100–125g shredded roast chicken (or two hard-boiled eggs), about 100g roasted carrots, some sauerkraut and a drizzle of pumpkin seed oil

After-Dinner Treat: A good-Gut Jelly and a mug of herbal tea

tip
Try adding torn nori sheets, a scrambled egg or a spoonful of coconut oil or ghee to your bone broth, or see page 116.

DAY 3

AM: 115–175ml hot water with lemon and 700ml–1 litre plain water with a pinch of sea salt

Breakfast: Reset variation of Power Parfait (see page 44), tea or coffee with 1 teaspoon coconut oil or ghee mixed in

Optional Mid-morning Probiotic Pick-me-up: 125–175ml kombucha or Fermented Fruit Soda (page 181)

Lunch: Green-leaf lettuce or baby spinach (as much as you like), 100–125g shredded roast chicken (or tinned sardines), about 150g roasted cauliflower, some sauerkraut, a squeeze of lemon juice, a drizzle of extra-virgin olive oil and a pinch each of cumin, salt and pepper

Snack: ½ avocado and some Raw Power Veggies (see page 42 – as much as you like)

Dinner: A bowl of bone broth with 100–150g of stir-fried veggies and an egg cooked in, a drizzle of tamari or coconut aminos, a dash of sesame or coconut oil, and a pinch of cayenne pepper (optional)

After Dinner Treat: A good-Gut Jelly and a mug of herbal tea

RESET REFLECTION

Now that you've completed your reset, let's take a few minutes to reflect on your experience:

♦ How did it go for you? Was anything challenging? Were some times of day or meals easier than others for you?

♦ Is there anything you want to bring into your normal everyday routine?

♦ Would you do this again? Would you change anything? (What response is your intuition giving you to this question?)

♦ How does your belly feel? Have there been any changes to your digestion? Energy? Mood?

Share one positive thing you learnt, felt or experienced using #gowithyourgutdiet!

HUNGRY FOR MORE?

I hope this reset has given you a taste for how healthy eating doesn't have to suck – and how it can actually be delicious and very satisfying. But no matter how it went (or didn't), I hope you are hungry for more and are ready to take the next step towards your healthiest you.

In the next chapter, I'm going to walk you through how to set yourself up for success in the kitchen every week and will share with you my top meal-prep tips, gut-healing kitchen-cupboard staples and superfoods. It is, after all, what you do most of the time that will have the biggest impact on your belly and your body.

My hope is that you will be feeling better after just three days, whether in terms of your energy levels, emotionally (you did something for you!) or physically. I suggest to many of my clients that they follow this gentle three-day meal plan once a season, or even once a month. I recommend that you take out your diary and schedule the next couple of times you plan to hit reset again. You could even invite a friend to do it with you!

tip

Not feeling totally 'reset' at the end of your three days? Feel free to keep going for an additional one to three days of gentle cleansing and see if you notice a difference then. You might also need a more customised plan for you: visit robynyoukilis. com/books for information on working with me.

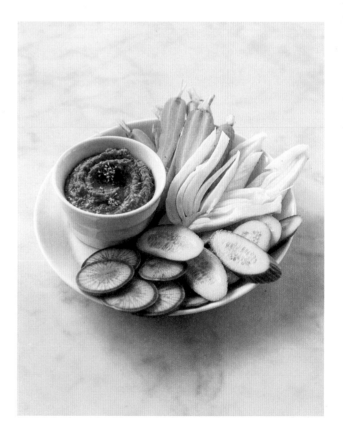

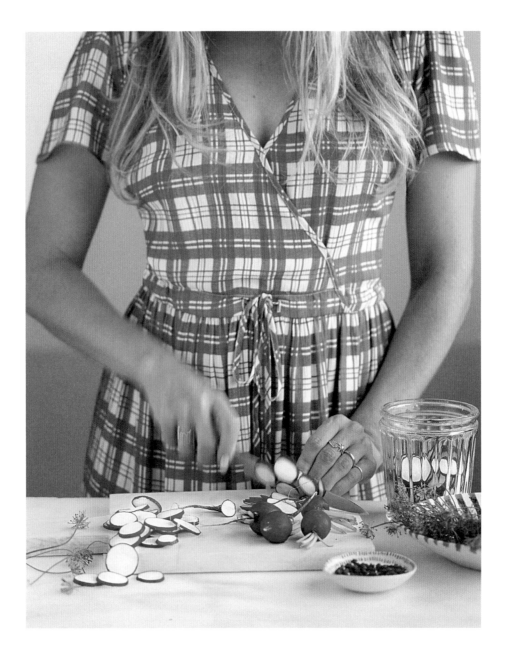

chapter five

LET'S GET COOKING

Here's the deal: home cooking is essential to weight loss. Cooking was the catalyst for so many changes in my body and life, and I'm confident that it can be for you, too!

Why is cooking for yourself such a big deal?

When you cook at home, you control the portions and proportions of foods on your plate and are able to load up on more of the nutrient-rich stuff (greens, healthy fats and quality protein) your body wants and needs. Even the best restaurants typically do not serve enough veggies. When I eat out, I have been known to order a nine-dollar side of kale because I know greens need to make up the majority of my plate, but it's taken me some time to get to that place, and it's not always easy to be the exception. Most people simply eat what's served to them, whether it's how they would build their plate at home or not.

In addition, when you make your own meals, you will often find you simplify your food and, by doing so, can hear more clearly the messages your gut is sending you about those foods. How can you expect to know what foods make you feel your best when you're not sure what's in your dinner because someone else has made it for you? It's hard! Cooking for yourself lets you take back control and feel empowered.

Finally, when you cook at home, you naturally end up eating more high-quality food without even thinking about it. When you're constantly eating out and grabbing food on the go, you're exposed to low-quality oils, processed starches and industrial farm-raised meat and fish. These foods can make you gain weight because your body doesn't break them down as efficiently as it does real, whole food.

HOW FAKE FOOD MESSES WITH YOUR GUT

Highly processed ingredients disrupt the natural balance of your gut bacteria and can make you feel bloated and sluggish. Many processed ingredients (including preservatives, fillers and chemicals) increase inflammation in your digestive system and damage your healthy gut bacteria. In one study, a college student ate strictly fast food (filled with those fake ingredients) for ten days. The result: his gut bacteria was devastated – about 40 per cent of the species were lost.

Additionally, processed ingredients interfere with your leptin and ghrelin levels, aka your hunger hormones. I know that hormones can feel like our enemies, but you need to know about these two important hormones and how they affect your metabolism and weight-loss goals. Your fat cells use leptin to tell the brain how much body fat they carry. Lots of leptin tells the brain that you have plenty of fat stored (and so don't need to eat), while low levels of leptin tell the brain that fat stores are low and that you are at risk of starvation (and so should eat). Ghrelin is a hormone made in the stomach that increases your appetite, particularly when you feel stressed. The production of ghrelin is supposed to drive you to eat, so you have the energy to handle whatever stressor is facing you.

When your leptin and ghrelin levels are thrown off, it's more difficult to know when you're hungry or full, and furthermore, if you're tired, thirsty, sad or happy. An imbalance in these hormones also causes inflammation and digestive issues.

The good news is that when you cook more of your food at home, you're exposed to a lot less of the fake stuff that messes with your body's natural state of health. Getting rid of what's getting in your body's way is a big step towards feeling your best.

Small shifts in how you approach cooking can make a huge difference in how you feel – a little time in the kitchen can have a big impact on your life. Even if you usually end with #PinterestFail dishes, anyone can do a little cooking. My stories, and so many of my clients' stories, are a testament to this:

'I came home tonight and felt inspired to cook up some chicken meatballs and zoodles (also new for me) and have a sit-down dinner – party of one. I decorated the space with a fresh flower and rose quartz to make it feel special!' – GRETA

'Also, this girl cleaned out her fridge and has started cooking with ease. I was really making everything way too hard – trapped in a spiral of my own resistance? Not every meal was perfect, but I'm annoyingly proud that I made eggs over-easy on the first try!' – MARGARET

I want cooking to feel stress-free and fun for you. In this chapter, I'll help you clean out your kitchen cupboards, then walk you through what to have on hand so that cooking this way becomes easy.

SET YOURSELF UP FOR SUCCESS IN THE KITCHEN

Have you ever searched through your wardrobe knowing that you have lots of clothes but finding nothing to wear? Consider for a moment that your kitchen cupboards might be set up this way, too – lots of old boxes of crackers, jars of who knows what and other mystery items that don't make a meal? When your fridge and cupboards are stocked with healthy options, you won't constantly have to weed through all the fluff to find the one thing that 'fits' – all the good stuff will be at your fingertips.

THE BIG CLEAR-OUT

It's time to go to work on a big blitz of your kitchen cupboards and keep only the foods that really light you up. Take everything out of your fridge and cupboards and off your shelves. You can do this one area at a time if that's easier, or go all out if you're feeling fired up.

You can't have mini chocolate brownies and packets of crisps in your face every day when you want to lose weight. No, these foods aren't necessarily off limits in the big scheme of life, but for now, they need to go. They're probably not the most supportive foods to have around on your journey.

Get rid of any foods that are a problem for you, then check the food labels and toss or donate anything containing the following ingredients:

- Sodium nitrite
- Hydrogenated or partially hydrogenated oils
- Refined palm oil
- Cottonseed oil
- Canola oil, soybean oil or vegetable oil
- BHA or BHT
- Margarine
- Hydrolyzed vegetable protein
- Parabens
- Artificial colours and/or flavours
- High-fructose corn syrup
- Caramel colouring
- Food dyes
- Sodium benzoate
- Aspartame
- Carrageenan
- Trans fats
- Splenda
- Equal
- Saccharin
- Monosodium glutamate (MSG)

'PROBLEM' FOODS

These are the foods that once you start eating, you can't stop. There's no concept of a serving with these foods (what, the whole bag isn't a serving?) and they often trigger other unhealthy habits. What foods are irresistible to you? Perhaps it's peanut butter. Do you struggle not to eat the whole jarful in one sitting? Or maybe it's toffee popcorn, granola or raw cashews. Do yourself a favour and keep these foods out of your home, at least for now. My guess is that you'll feel lighter by simply not having these options within reach.

Toss packaged and processed foods and anything with a long list of fake ingredients. These foods damage your microbiome and mess with your hunger hormones.

You can use this clean-out time to reflect on what's going on beneath the surface that's keeping you from your goal weight. You probably know the biggest habit that needs to go before you can lose those extra kilos. If it was just about eating more piles of steamed greens and drinking water, no one would have an issue with gut health or stubborn belly weight.

WHAT ABOUT FLOUR AND SUGAR?

I'm not specifically asking you to ditch white flour or sugar, because I'm less concerned about you having these ingredients on your shelves than I am with those ready-to-eat foods that are so hard to resist. If you want to make your auntie's famous chocolate cake once or twice a year with that white flour and white sugar, go for it. I'd prefer you to focus on clearing out those ready-to-eat foods that don't support your gut or your mind in making the best choices on daily basis.

DO YOU SHARE YOUR KITCHEN?

If you share a kitchen, this clear-out may be a little trickier. I recommend having a conversation with your husband/partner/roommate before you toss his or her beloved cheese puffs. Explain to them why you are doing this and keep the focus on you. Maybe you can agree to keep the foods you don't want to be eating on a certain shelf or in a basket. In fact, a study undertaken by Cornell University shows that people are much more likely to eat the foods they can see, so if there are foods you want to avoid and you can't throw them away, hide them away at the back of a shelf and give your husband/partner/roommate the map!

STOCK YOUR KITCHEN

Once you've cleared out the junk, the list opposite is a great place to start when you're stocking a healthy kitchen. You can always adjust staples to your taste, but if you're new to the healthy cooking and eating game, use this list to help take out some of the guesswork.

This isn't a weekly shopping list but rather a helpful guide to give you an idea of the fresh produce, frozen items and kitchen-cupboard staples I have on hand most of the time. The list is organised by where I store these must-have items. For example, you don't necessarily find sourdough bread in the refrigerator section, but this is where I keep mine for optimal freshness.

tip

Choose organic versions of these staples whenever possible and always go for GMO-free.

STOCKING YOUR KITCHEN

Fridge

- Light leafy greens (e.g. rocket, red leaf lettuce and baby spinach)
- Dark leafy greens (e.g. kale, Swiss chard and spring greens)
- Spiralised or 'riced' vegetables
- Root vegetables (carrots, beetroot, parsnips, sweet potatoes and others)
- Raw Power Veggies (celery, jicama, radishes and fennel)
- Eggs
- Tempeh
- Grass-fed butter and ghee
- Sauerkraut and fermented vegetables (raw and unpasteurised)
- Kombucha, kefir or kvass
- Coconut water
- Apple juice or cider (no added sweetener)
- Local fermented breads (like sourdough or miche)
- Unsweetened non-dairy milk (almond, coconut or flax)
- Natural yogurt
- Matcha powder (ceremonial grade)

Freezer

- Wild fish (e.g. salmon, trout and cod)
- Veggie burgers
- Veggies of all kinds, including 'riced' vegetables
- Berries
- Cooked grains
- Portions of homemade soups and sauces, frozen in containers
- Gluten-free, sprouted breads (purchased from the fridge or freezer section)
- Dark chocolate
- Favourite raw nuts and seeds (see tip)

Kitchen cupboards

- Tins of small fish and seafood (e.g. wild sardines, wild salmon and smoked oysters)
- Tins of tuna or mackerel
- Canned or dried beans (chickpeas, black, cannellini and lentils)
- Bean, quinoa or brown rice pastas
- Tins of chopped tomatoes (no added sugar)
- Rolled oats
- Dry grains (quinoa, millet and amaranth)
- Onions, shallots and garlic
- Vegetable or chicken stock
- Nut and seed butters (almond butter, peanut butter, tahini and coconut butter)
- Gluten-free, low-sugar granola
- Simple-ingredient energy bars
- Selection of teas
- Quality sea salt and black pepper
- Favourite spices and dried herbs
- Nutritional yeast
- Apple cider vinegar
- Gluten-free soy sauce, tamari or coconut aminos
- Oils (olive oil, coconut oil and avocado oil)
- A variety of seaweed (nori, dulse and snacks)
- Chia seeds
- Dried fruit (e.g. figs, dates and goji berries)
- Collagen peptides
- Psyllium husk
- Aloe vera juice

tip

Nuts and seeds are susceptible to mould and toxins. Storing them in the fridge or freezer keeps them fresh, which means they'll be less likely to cause belly issues. For this reason, I like buying these items in small quantities from the bulk bins in busy shops.

MY FAVORITE GUT RESET FOODS

	GUT-HEALING PROPERTIES	WEIGHT-LOSS PROPERTIES	RECIPES/ USES
RAW, FERMENTED SAUERKRAUT	One of the best natural sources of probiotics. Adding 1–3 tablespoons to your plate at every meal will help rebalance your microbiome.	Eating fermented foods, like sauerkraut, can help curb cravings, especially sugar cravings, making it easier to stick to your weight-loss goals.	See pages 56–7 for more on sauerkraut, including my favourite ways to eat it!
BONE BROTH	Full of collagen and gelatin, which help reduce inflammation in the gut and promote balance of gut bacteria.	Bone broth is rich in protein and amino acids, which help you feel full and satisfied longer.	Drink a mug of broth for a nutrient-rich snack, use it as the base for soups (such as those on pages 105, 113 and 116) or cook grains or veggies in it.
BITTER GREENS	Bitter greens (e.g. dandelion, mustard, escarole, rocket and the tops of root veggies such as beetroot, turnips and radishes) are naturally detoxifying and cleansing for your gut.	One of my favourite teachers, Paul Pitchford, says, 'Bitter foods, sweet life.' Our current diets tend to be so oversweetened that bitter is a taste our bodies are craving.	Try my Honeymoon Greens (see page 153), Healing Greens Soup (see page 112), Blueberry and Rocket Salad (see page 98), Smoked Trout and Lentil Salad (see page 102).
YOGURT	Natural yogurt is rich in gut-healing probiotics. Not everyone can eat dairy, so it's great that there are coconut- and nut-based options that also provide lots of healthy bacteria your gut needs (see page 29).	Yogurt is also packed with protein. I find that when I eat a protein-rich breakfast, I'm full for longer and have fewer cravings throughout the day.	Use in Power Parfait (see pages 36–7) and in place of sour cream in most recipes. Try my Blueberry Chia Muffins (see page 85) and Superwoman Bread (see page 95).
COLLAGEN	Collagen is the most abundant protein in our bodies. It helps strengthen the gut lining and is great for skin, hair and nail health – the 'glue' that helps hold our body together.	Protein is a macronutrient that is essential for weight loss and helps you stay full for hours after a meal. Collagen is a pure form of easily digestible protein.	You can buy a grass-fed powder and mix it into your morning beverage (e.g. my Magical Morning Matcha, see page 184), blend it into a smoothie or use it anywhere you'd use protein powder.

	GUT-HEALING PROPERTIES	WEIGHT-LOSS PROPERTIES	RECIPES/ USES
TEMPEH	Tempeh is naturally fermented and therefore a great gut-healing option, especially if you're vegetarian or simply want to take a break from meat.	Not only is tempeh rich in protein, but it also contains niacin and riboflavin, which help boost your metabolism.	I love to simply sear tempeh in coconut oil and gluten-free soy sauce. You can also try my Savoury Sunflower Butter Tempeh (see page 137).
ROOT VEGETABLES	Root veggies are super calming for the gut. For example, sweet potatoes have anti-inflammatory properties and beetroot is known to soothe indigestion.	Root veggies reduce cravings for white carbs since they're naturally starchy and they lessen sugar cravings because they're sweet.	Roast a big tray of root veggies to have on hand for your Good Gut Rule of Five meals all week.
FERMENTED DRINKS	Fermented drinks, like fermented foods, pack a powerful punch of gut-friendly probiotics and offer a unique variety of different strains.	Many fermented drinks are naturally sweet and carbonated, making them healthier alternatives to soda or energy drinks.	Try my Fermented Fruit Soda (see page 181), Pineapple Tepache (see page 183) and Kombucha Cocktail (see page 188).
FENNEL	Think of fennel as a highly nutritious, more digestible version of cabbage that can decrease bloating (rather than cause it). This veggie is highly recommended for those with IBS.	Snacking on fennel (as you would on celery or carrots) is an easy way to add more veggies and crowd out junkier snacks. Plus, it really helps curb sugar cravings since it's so naturally sweet.	Crunch on it raw or try it in Go with Your Gut Lemonade (see page 180), Three-Seed Tea (see page 183), Cleansing Fennel Salad (see page 101), Kale Spanakopita (see page 127) and Veggie-Packed Meatballs (page 125).
GHEE	Ghee is easier to digest than butter since it's nearly lactose-free. It also contains butyric acid, which supports the health and healing of the small intestine.	Fat won't make you fat! It's necessary to include healthy fats in your diet for proper nutrient absorption and satiety.	Use ghee anywhere you'd use butter or coconut oil – probably about half the recipes in this book!

TEN CREATIVE WAYS TO USE PROBIOTIC-RICH SAUERKRAUT

1. Toss it into a salad

2. Upgrade your avocado toast

3. Throw it into an omelette in the last 30 seconds of cooking

4. Stir it into your hummus to add more tang

5. Mix it into guacamole

6. Add it as a topping on healthy homemade pizza after you take it out of the oven

7. Add it to Spring Green Salad Wraps (see page 100)

8. Use it instead of pickles on a burger

9. Chop it up and add it to tuna or chicken salad instead of relish

10. Mix it into any slaw

MY LOVE AFFAIR WITH SAUERKRAUT

Sauerkraut is hands down my favourite superfood. If you're going to pick one food from the previous list, sauerkraut has to be it. Is there anything sauerkraut can't do? It strengthens your immune system and provides essential B vitamins (especially B12). Plus, it will help you to curb sugar cravings and balance your gut bacteria. Sauerkraut is also high in antioxidants, which can help protect your body from developing chronic diseases.

But the number one reason I love sauerkraut is for its flavour. Sauerkraut comes in all different varieties and is an easy way to add a serious flavour punch to a meal.

Fresh sauerkraut is worlds apart from what you might have tried slopped on a street-stand hot dog (which is always the tinned variety). Raw, fermented sauerkraut has a bright, almost lemony tanginess that's refreshing, but not sharp. When serving up a dish, think of sauerkraut as you would a squeeze of lemon or other acid. Sauerkraut (and its juice) adds a zing that brightens up any meal.

You can start by buying naturally fermented sauerkraut at the supermarket or deli. It will be in the refrigerated section and the only ingredients should be cabbage, salt and herbs or spices like caraway seeds and turmeric. There may also be another vegetable or two.

Fermented foods, like sauerkraut, are an essential part of the Good Gut Rule of Five plate, so you'll want to experiment with adding these foods to your everyday meals.

I've even heard you can blend it into smoothies, although I haven't tried that myself yet!

Buying sauerkraut is a good first step, but once you've got used to it, you can take things to the next level – in terms of both flavour and gut health – by making your own. You can find my tried-and-true recipe for sauerkraut, which has a fiery flavour zing, in my first book, *Go with Your Gut*, or at robynyoukilis.com/books.

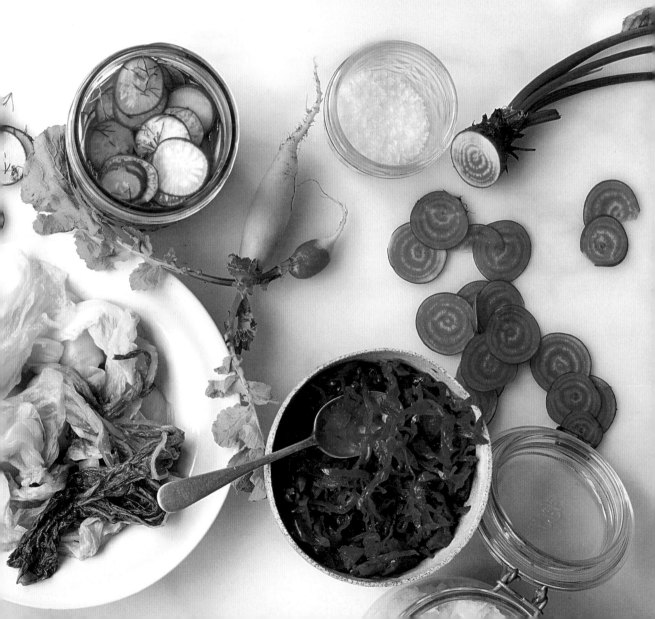

SPARKLE UP WITH SUPPLEMENTS

They say that diamonds are a girl's best friend, and I'm all for the sparkly, fun stuff, so think of supplements as the little diamonds that help your insides shine. Our nutritional needs are always changing and so it's good to have some extra support.

The following are some supplement options that are supportive of your gut-health and weight-loss goals. I recommend that you try one or two from this list and see how you feel and, because supplementation is such a personal thing, that you seek the advice of a health coach or doctor if you have any questions or hesitations before beginning this, or any other, new regime.

♦ **Digestive enzymes** help you break down your food more efficiently. They add more of the natural enzymes your body produces to digest your food. Take these before meals, and especially when you're dining out or find yourself eating anything that could be troublesome for your body to digest.

♦ **Probiotics** fast-track your microbiome to be its best self. You can get probiotics from dietary sources like sauerkraut and kombucha, but it's great to take a daily dose in pill form as well (especially when following my Good Gut Reset plan). I recommend cycling your probiotic supplement to ensure you're getting a broad range of bacteria strains.

♦ **L-glutamine** is key for healing leaky gut and boosting absorption. It can repair damage to your intestinal lining by filling in the gaps that occur from undiagnosed celiac, toxins and stress. (Head back to page 19 for more on leaky gut and other digestive disorders.)

♦ **Liquorice root** (aka DGL) is my gut-healing candy! Not only is it soothing for your belly, DGL helps balance cortisol levels, which makes it especially beneficial if your gut issues have any connected emotional component (and let's be honest, whose don't?). Plus, if you like the flavour of licorice, this supplement tastes just like sweeties!

♦ **Aloe vera** is a great go-to if you aren't sure what's going on with your belly but something doesn't feel quite right. It's soothing and calming. Imagine it cooling any internal sunburn (inflammation) that may be going on inside the body. Plus, it helps you poop.

♦ **Psyllium husk** is my secret weapon for clients who just can't go for number twos (or those who can go, but for whom it doesn't feel easy or complete). Psyllium husk is the main ingredient in Metamucil. It's made from the husk of a plant and it's pure soluble fibre. It promotes easy elimination by pulling waste out of the colon more quickly and efficiently. I also love psyllium husk because it's a prebiotic food.

♦ **Magnesium** is calming for your nerves, muscles and digestive tract. It helps with bowel movements in a really gentle way. For most people, magnesium has a calming effect, but I've had a few clients who are more stimulated by it.

disclaimer

Supplements are personal to your body's needs. If you are currently taking any medication, are pregnant or nursing, or have a serious medical condition, please consult with your doctor before beginning to take any new supplements.

SUPERFOODS AND ADAPTOGENS

Superfoods are nutrient-dense foods that are high in antioxidants, polyphenols, vitamins and minerals. Really, any whole food can be classified as a superfood, but here I'm talking about the extra-special ones that specifically help with your gut-health and weight-loss goals. Adaptogens help your body adapt to stress. This means you'll stay in the parasympathetic state more often – key for weight loss and a good gut.

If the idea of a superfood doesn't feel right for you, feel free to skip this section for now.

These are some of my favourite superfoods for gut health and weight loss:

♦ **Chia seeds** add bulk to your digestive tract and help with good poops. They create a gelatinous mass that passes through your intestines and cleans up old waste and toxins on its way out.

♦ **Spirulina and chlorella** calm inflammation in the body and cool off stress flare-ups. You can simply add them to your smoothies or mix with water.

♦ **Goji berries** have been used in traditional Chinese medicine since around 200 BCE for their ability to generate feelings of well-being, support gut health, help build stronger muscles and improve cardiovascular health.

♦ **Ashwagandha** is one of the key adaptogens that helps your body respond to stress. Add ¼ teaspoon to your Magical Morning Matcha (page 184) or smoothie to help stay centred and slim. Relaxation is key to losing weight and keeping any gut flare-ups or constipation at bay. Plus ashwagandha gives you a serious concentration boost.

♦ **Matcha** is another favourite adaptogen for weight loss because it gives you a boost without caffeine or sugar. It also helps balance hormones, which is important in shedding those extra pounds. Oh, and it's great for your libido, too!

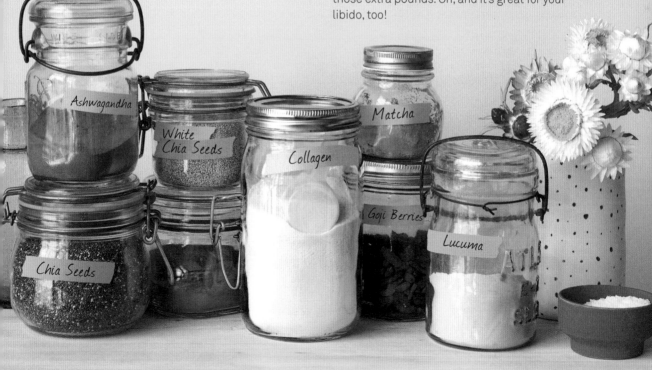

BUILD YOUR PERFECT PLATE

Your kitchen is now well stocked – so what's next? How do you take all these ingredients and turn them into dinner?

Of course, you could cook every meal from scratch, but I'm guessing you won't want to or won't have time to.

I'm a firm believer that a little planning is the first step to getting the right foods on your plate. Contrary to what many believe, meal prep doesn't have to feel like a scary thing that other people are capable of but you aren't. You don't have to do it all at once or lose half your weekend, and, yes, it can even be fun. With the right amount of preparation, assembling your plate according to the Good Gut Rule of Five becomes easy.

tip

A great question to ask yourself when you're considering your meal is this: how can I make it just 10 per cent better? Could you use extra-virgin olive oil instead of a processed vegetable oil? Could you upgrade to organic the next time you go grocery shopping? Could you add sauerkraut? Would your tummy feel better if you left out the cheese just for today?

For a quick review on the Good Gut Rule of Five – these are the five components you should include in your lunches and dinners:

1 Greens

2 Healthy Fat

3 Protein

4 Fermented Food

5 Cooked Vegetable

MEAL PREP FOR SUCCESS

For many of my clients, learning my easy way of meal prepping is 'life-changing'. One of my clients, Gannon, is a perfect example of what I'm talking about: 'I meal prepped last night and feel so at ease knowing what I'm going to eat every day, loving what I'm eating and confident that my fridge has enough food in it for the next week.' This is what meal prep is all about – having the foods you actually want to be eating ready for you and feeling the ease and support that comes from that.

YOUR MEAL PREP GAME PLAN

Let me walk you through exactly how to start meal prepping so you have the components of your perfect plate ready to go when you are.

Here are the basics you'll need for each week.

This list may look familiar – if you've done the Good Gut Reset (see pages 39–47), you've alraedy had a taste of what my meal prep game plan looks like. That was the point!

If you can't commit to this whole list right away, feel free to start with just one item from the list and build from there.

1 Roast a tray (or ideally two) of vegetables

I always try to prepare one hearty, starchy veggie, such as sweet potato or winter squash, and one other cooked vegetable, such as Brussels sprouts, broccoli or cauliflower.

Preheat the oven to 220°C/ gas mark 7. Chop your veggies of choice into equal-sized pieces, or as close as you can get. Arrange them in one layer on a baking tray. Toss to coat with melted ghee or coconut or avocado oil and then sprinkle with salt and pepper. Roast for 25–45 minutes, until tender all the way through and slightly browned, flipping once during the cooking process. Store in glass containers (check out my favourites in my online shop at robynyoukilis.com/books).

2 Wash and prep your greens

The difference between me eating greens and not eating greens is having them washed, chopped and ready to go. Yes, you can buy prewashed and chopped bags of greens, but fresh is best (for taste and nutrition). Additionally, many bitter greens (see My Favourite Gut Reset Foods on page 54) need an extra rinse to remove stubborn grit, so you're less likely to find them in your grocer's prewashed section. You might as well buy yourself a salad spinner and make this a part of your weekly routine.

Put the greens in a big bowl and fill with water. Use your hands to shake the leaves about in the water, then transfer the leaves to the salad spinner. Drain the water, rinse out any grit at the bottom of the bowl and give the greens another dunk if needed. Spin the leaves dry in the salad spinner, or lay them out on a clean tea-towel and pat them dry. Chop the leaves and store in reusable produce bags with some kitchen paper (to absorb excess moisture).

WHOLE GRAINS?

If your family runs on carbs (I know my husband does!), make a big batch of a whole grain (quinoa, rice, barley, farro, etc.) at the beginning of the week, too. I use my rice cooker – perfect quinoa every time! Alternatively, you can buy precooked rice in most supermarkets these days.

3 Prep one or two proteins of choice

I always have at least one or two easy ready-to-eat proteins in my fridge or kitchen cupboards. I've included a few ideas here: some are recipes and some are quicker, precooked options.

Easy protein recipes:
- Roast chicken – either roast it yourself or you buy one from the supermarket. But do check the label for other ingredients: it should have only olive oil, lemon and natural herbs listed – no preservatives, margarine or ingredients you can't pronounce. Visit robynyoukilis.com/books to download my simple whole roasted chicken recipe.
- Seared tempeh
- Hard-boiled eggs
- The Simplest Salmon (see page 124)
- Grilled shrimp
- Veggie-Packed Meatballs (see page 125)

Precooked or grab-and-go options:
- Smoked salmon
- Veggie burgers
- Tinned fish, such as tuna or mackerel, sardines, smoked trout and oysters (buy BPA-free tins)

4 Make one or two tasty dressings or condiments

Dressings and condiments can take meals to another level of deliciousness! You can use them in salads and grain bowls or to accompany a simple piece of fish and roasted veggies. Try the following recipes:

- Homemade Honey Mustard (see page 98)
- Roasted Shallot Vinaigrette (see page 102)
- Beetroot Hummus (see page 148)
- Amped-Up Ketchup (see page 132)

5 Make a batch of Power Parfaits

As I mentioned in chapter 3, my Power Parfait was the game-changer for me after I had my daughter, and I get messages every day on how this yummy breakfast has transformed mornings for others, too.

6 Stock your snacks and treats

Well-planned snacks can keep your blood sugar balanced and prevent a binge. Here are some suggestions of snacks to keep on hand:

- Hard-boiled eggs (make and peel them in advance, then season with salt, pepper and Italian seasoning)
- Healthy protein bars (again, check ingredients and choose the ones with the least grams of sugar)
- Half an avocado eaten with a spoon straight out of its skin
- Sliced organic, nitrate- and carrageenan-free cold meats, wrapped in a nori sheet
- Small tub of natural yogurt
- Small slice of organic cheese
- Apple or celery slices with a single serving of almond butter
- Raw fennel slices
- Single-serving packet of raw nuts
- Good-Gut Jellies (see page 165)

tip

I keep psyllium husk and apple juice on hand so I can always have a batch of my Good Gut Gellies (page 165) in the fridge. These Gellies are the perfect evening snack – they satisfy that sweet tooth while giving you plenty of gut-friendly fiber that will help ensure you go first thing in the morning the next day.

YOUR NEW SAVING GRACE

Let me help make meal prep happen for you.

First, get clear on when you can make time to get yourself into the kitchen. Ideally, take out your calendar now and look at the rest of this week and next. Sunday afternoon and evening are the most popular times for meal prep, but if you're like me and you travel a lot at weekends, you may want to set aside time on Monday, or even Tuesday, or do some of this in parts throughout the week. Think about what works best for you and your life. Grab your workbook and write down when you are going to meal prep.

Next, are there any kitchen tools you need to buy to facilitate your meal prep process? Do you have storage containers, reusable veggie bags, lunch boxes for any meals that need assembling in advance? Do you want to invest in a rice cooker?

Where and when are you going to buy your food? Do you need to schedule a trip to the supermarket or farmers' market? Are there any speciality items or superfoods you'll need to order online?

If the very thought of making a trip to the supermarket makes you feel exhausted, I suggest you look into grocery delivery services. Between running my business and being a mum, I find it's worth the small delivery fee for me to have my groceries brought to my doorstep.

Finally, how can you make your meal-prep time more fun? Do you need to download a podcast or audiobook, or throw on an awesome playlist? Would it help to have a cute apron to wear, or a new set of dishes?

DON'T GO NUTS

I've said it before, and I'll likely say it in every book I write: nuts are not popcorn! Nuts are not something to eat by the handful. Notice how they come from trees in those hard-to-crack shells? That's because nature didn't intend for us to gobble them up in large quantities! Nowadays, they're almost too easily available – in nut butter form, shelled and in bulk – and since they're so delicious, we tend to overeat them. They are healthy, but only if eaten in moderation. For this reason, I recommend buying single-serving packages of nuts, or serving them in small single-serving ramekins or other small dishes.

I get that meal prep may not be glamorous, catchy, or cover-of-the-magazine cute. It's about getting in the kitchen and getting your hands and baking sheets dirty (schedule your manicure for the next day!). But the results are worth it. Think of that OMG moment when you open your fridge and it's full of foods that are ready to go when you are. It's the best feeling!

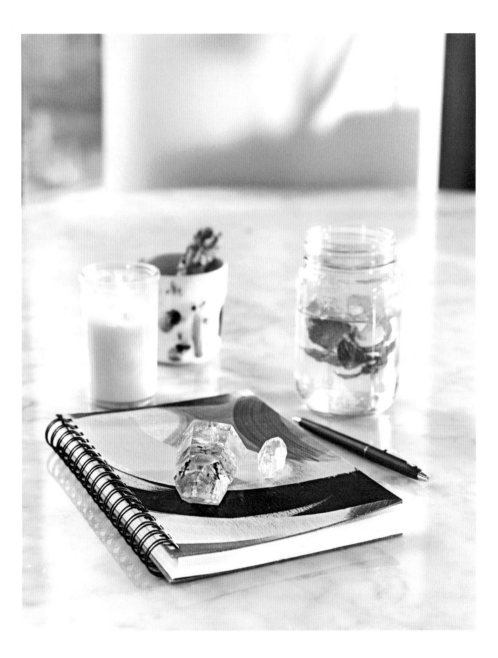

chapter six

FINDING YOUR INTUITIVE FOOD VOICE

Thus far, we've talked a lot about what to eat. How you can eat is just as important, if not more.

Your body is not designed to digest food if you're stressed or distracted. In chapter 3 (see page 33), we learnt that your body has two main states: rest and digest (parasympathetic) and fight or flight (sympathetic). You are physically not able to be in both stages at once. If you are stressed out while eating (or right after you eat), your body can't digest your food, which leads to weight gain and poor digestion.

You're better equipped to connect with your intuitive food voice and your body's natural hunger and satiety signals when you are present with your meals. When you tune in, you'll hear the signals your gut is sending you – when it's hungry and when it's full.

What if 'mindful eating' just doesn't seem to happen in your day-to-day life? You have e-mails to respond to, kids to drop off and pick up, friends to call and the list goes on. While eating mindfully seems like a good idea in theory, it's not something that you can bring down into your reality.

I get it. I knew about the benefits of mindful eating for years before my daily practice finally clicked into place. How did I do it?

In my coaching practice, Your Healthiest You, I developed my 123 Food Freedom Tool, and this three-step process to mindful eating was featured in my first book, *Go with Your Gut*. The 123 Food Freedom Tool will help you slow down at meal times, enjoy your food more and say goodbye to annoying digestive issues like bloating and heartburn.

A MINDFUL EATING PROGRAM

I'm including this tool here again because it's so foundational. It's one of the best ways to transform your eating experience without actually changing any of the foods on your plate.

My 456 Eat and Complete Practice is the next phase in my approach to shedding extra kilos that aren't you. I like to think of this as my post-meal meditation. This practice will help you drop into your parasympathetic nervous system, get clear on which foods are serving you and address any emotional issues that may be causing you to overeat.

If you've been using the 123 Food Freedom Tool, you can add the 456 Eat and Complete Practice right away. You can also start using both of them and you'll notice a huge difference in how you feel in your body.

You've heard about intuition, right? This magical thing that's meant to guide us? Well, your intuitive food voice is what your gut (all those bacteria in your physical gut and your intuitive gut instinct) is telling you to eat and what to avoid.

'It's incredible what just a few days of changing your habits can do for you. Not only do I feel healthier in my body, but I feel clearer in my mind – I've been more productive at work! I'm also more in tune with my body and what it wants. I went to this health food store yesterday and browsed through the 'healthy' snacks and chocolates. Usually, I would crack and buy something but yesterday I heard a clear 'no' from my gut and I listened and I walked away. It was actually easy!' – MAUD

THE 123 FOOD FREEDOM TOOL

♦ Step 1: Look

When was the last time you allowed your eyes to take in the experience of eating? Eating is a complete sensory experience, and if we don't include one of our most vital senses – our sight – we are out of touch with the idea that we have eaten. Next time you're about to consume something, take a moment to feast your eyes on it. Yes, you'll want to do this with the beautiful recipes you make from this book (for example the Smoked Trout and Lentil Salad on page 102), but make it a habit with simple snacks and less exciting, on-the-go bites, too.

♦ Step 2: Breathe

Before you take your first bite, take a deep belly breath or two. Taking a good, deep breath brings you into the present and into your body again (which is necessary because you're about to use your body to eat). Feel your belly expand and release and the gentle 'ahhh' that comes with that simple action.

♦ Step 3: Chew

Chewing is so important that I've created an entire free online coaching programme around this practice. You can join us any time at www.thechewingchallenge.com. The goal? To chew each mouthful completely (i.e. until it becomes liquid) before swallowing. When you chew your food thoroughly, you stimulate your digestive juices to better process your meal. In addition, you'll naturally slow down and so will probably eat a little less.

THE 456 EAT AND COMPLETE PRACTICE

♦ Step 4: Rest and Digest

After you've used your 123 Food Freedom Tool at a meal or snack time, it's time to digest. This means spending an extra minute or two or ten (the more the better) sitting with your empty plate or bowl after you've completed your meal, just taking that moment to breathe and be.

I know that finding real time to eat may already be a stretch, so asking for an additional minute might feel completely unattainable, but you can shift your mind-set from 'There's no way' to 'I am going to try'. It actually takes about twenty minutes for your body to register that it's full, so it's important to give your gut time to send those full signals to your brain so you aren't jumping out of your seat to help yourself to seconds that you aren't really hungry for.

♦ Step 5: Mark the End

You wouldn't write a sentence without punctuation and you shouldn't leave a meal without marking the end. Maybe just take a deep belly breath to say thanks: to your food, your body for digesting it or whoever cooked it – even if that's yourself.

You can also mark the end of a meal by clearing the table, putting leftovers away and washing dishes. If someone else is on washing-up duty (lucky you), make a cup of digestion-friendly tea – Three-Seed Tea (see page 185).

♦ Step 6: Pause and Reflect

The last step in the 456 Eat and Complete Practice is to notice how you feel. Are you still hungry, satisfied or overly full? What's going on in your brain? Are you judging yourself for what you just ate? Take a minute to feel what's going on in your body and become conscious of the experience between you and your food.

FINDING YOUR INTUITIVE FOOD VOICE

We're fed so much information about diet and lifestyle trends that it's easy to get confused and stuck under the layers of opinions out there, whether it's what *Vogue* magazine recommending what to eat, your best friend's latest diet or what your yoga instructor thinks about smoothies and juices.

You can learn the recipes, the tools and the tricks, but this will never become part of you until you learn to listen to your own body, to connect to your own inner guru, your own intuitive voice.

This inner knowing is what takes the power away from the birthday cake, the third glass of wine or whatever 'problem' food you're trying not to eat. This is your internal compass that will steer you back to you. Check in, again and again and again.

The 123 Food Freedom Tool and 456 Eat and Complete Practice will help you slow down and connect to your own intuitive food voice. (I promise, it's in there!)

I highly recommend writing down what you notice in a journal. Not only will this strengthen your intuitive food voice, but you'll also have a paper trail to reflect on. From this you can identify any foods or situations that aren't serving your gut health and weight-loss efforts.

Also, if you're sipping tea and writing in your journal, you're less likely to go hunting through the cabinets for chocolate or those cookies you know you just can't stop eating.

HOW TO FOOD-MOOD JOURNAL

Over the next two weeks, take stock of which foods make you feel fabulous, and which don't.

Grab a little notebook and after each meal (or at the end of the day), jot down how you're feeling. Focusing on how you feel is an easy way to check in. Use specific 'feeling words' that help you understand your body state, such as centered, focused, fulfilled, tired, annoyed, jittery, or happy.

Keep your journal close by to note when you have a strong positive or negative physical, mental, or emotional reaction to a certain food or food combination. You may feel fine right after a meal but later feel bloated and moody.

For example . . .

- Do you crash soon after your afternoon sweet treat?
- Do steamed sweet potatoes make you feel calm and energised?
- Is your daily glass of wine (or two) totally draining your energy the next morning?
- Does gluten make your tummy feel all funny and unsettled?

Don't forget to track your 'wins', too! If you have eaten roasted squash with your evening meal and notice you're sleeping deeper, great! If you suspect that your salads are not filling enough, i.e. you still want a bag of pretzels at 2 p.m., make note of this and make a bigger portion next time. Check whether you've followed the Good Gut Rule of Five, too

◇

DON'T FORGET TO TRACK YOUR 'WINS', TOO!

———

You can also use your Food-Mood Journal to reflect on other habits or factors that may be helping (or hurting) your weight-loss goals. Is it easier to feel satisfied by your lunch when you take it outside? Are you able to skip that second glass of wine if you take a minute for yourself when you get home from work? Or maybe you find yourself with a stomach ache every time you have dinner with a certain friend, or finishing off a jar of almond butter every time you've checked at your bank statement?

These are just a few examples of what you might uncover as you observe your body, but they're just that – examples. Perhaps everything I've mentioned is the exact opposite for you. The more you practise checking in, the easier it will be to identify the foods that support you best.

@ *Download your free Food-Mood Journal template at robynyoukilis.com/ books.*

A NEW BREED OF BALANCE

How many times have you heard someone say, 'Just eat a balanced diet'? But the big question is, how do you know you've finally landed in this heavenly realm of balance? So many of us are striving so hard to find a sense of balance in our food and our lives, but it almost feels like we can never quite get there. Why? Because we're constantly comparing ourselves to other people. You, your BFF, your mom, and that girl you follow on social media all have different needs for a balanced diet.

For example, some of us can handle some processed foods and caffeinated drinks while others can't. Some of us do well with animal proteins, some of us don't. It's about finding your definition of balance and sticking to rituals that keep you anchored to your intuitive food voice. This is how you know when your body can handle that amazing homemade upgraded Strawberry Shortcake (page 170), and when it needs a big plate of steamed kale drizzled with pumpkin seed oil. It's about checking in with your gut instead of ignoring it and grabbing whatever everyone else is.

You may think your intuitive food voice only wants pizza and peanut butter cups (or peanut butter cups ON pizza?), but I promise it has more wisdom than that. It's time to stop comparing and despairing, and start using and trusting your gut to find your definition of balance.

BECOMING A WELLNESS BABE

What keeps us from feeling happy and at home in our bodies, regardless of the number on the scale, are the heavy thoughts of what *used to be*. A dress size. A diet. An ex-boyfriend. An old job. Holding on to that *used to be* mind-set will keep you feeling stuck no matter how much progress you've made.

When my client Eliza came to me, she was in a rut. She was frustrated with food in general and felt like she couldn't get back to her "old self" no matter what she tried.

I reached out to Robyn because I wanted to learn how to take better care of my body. There are so many fad diets and confusing messages out there, it's hard to know what to believe.

After working with her I got back to basics in the best way possible. I now eat the foods that make me feel good, not what I think I 'should' eat according to someone else's plan. And guess what? It works. I do feel good. I feel lighter and happier.

I've definitely lost physical weight (maybe 5 to 10 pounds? I no longer weigh myself!), but it's so much more than that—it's the 'emotional weight' that was bogging me down. I didn't try to lose weight or count calories, but instead I focused on nourishing my gut and nurturing myself every single day.

— ELIZA

Eliza is my definition of a wellness babe. Her biggest transformation wasn't that she was able to fit in her size whatever jeans again, but that she discovered a new, even more brilliant version of herself.

Just as with Eliza, your body will naturally adjust to crave the foods that are best for you as your intuitive food voice strengthens. It will no longer be an excruciating decision-making process. More and more you'll just know.

Becoming a wellness babe is about knowing what makes you feel good now. It's about identifying your hell yes's and your no thank you's. It's about continually checking in and knowing when you can say, 'I'll have what she's having' and when you affirm, 'This is what I need today'. It's about getting clearer and clearer on what you want in your life and soaring from that place of intuition.

And that is how you become 'thin from within'. It all begins with you.

Love your guts,
Robyn

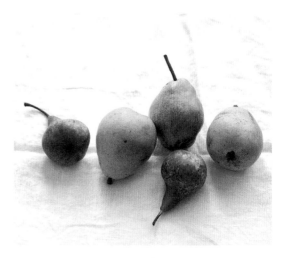

INTO THE KITCHEN

◇

NOW IT'S TIME FOR
THE EXTRA FUN PART:
THE RECIPES!

_____

My entire journey into health and wellness started because of my deep love of food.

Any way you slice it, **food equals love.**

Whatever challenges, struggles or confusion you've had with cooking and food, the bottom line is that food is a way we show love and also how we receive it. I grew up in a home where this was all too true. My mum always cooked delicious meals for our family – as I've mentioned, Coq au Vin was a regular Wednesday night dinner in our home. Her food was infused with love. I bonded with my dad over giant soft pretzels, and my brother and I had a ritual of getting vanilla coke floats together.

If you want to look or feel a certain way, you must get in the driver's seat of your life and you must get in the kitchen.

We've talked about all the ways home cooking supports your gut-health and weight-loss goals – when you cook for yourself, you can eat more of the good stuff and control the ratio and portions of the foods on your plate (hello Good Gut Rule of Five!) You also naturally end up with more high-quality foods, as well as fewer processed foods (which throw off the delicate balance of your gut bacteria and sabotage your weight-loss goals), when you cook at home. But the most important reason of all to cook is the simple fact that there's no better way to sharpen your intuition than by getting creative in the kitchen.

Whether you're completely at home roasting trays of veggies in your oven, or whether you currently use it as a place to store pots and pans, I encourage you to approach cooking the recipes in this book as a fun, messy and delicious challenge!

It's time to drop the pressure of perfectionism and pick up the fork of pure pleasure and dive in!

Let's eat!

◇

IF YOU WANT TO LOOK
OR FEEL A CERTAIN WAY,
YOU MUST GET IN THE
DRIVER'S SEAT OF YOUR
LIFE AND YOU MUST GET
IN THE KITCHEN.

THE
RECIPES

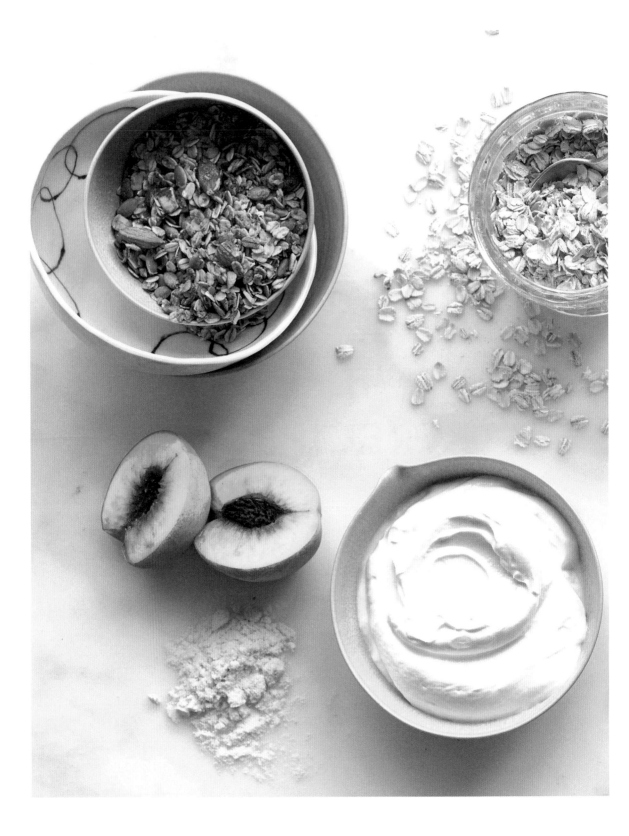

◇

MORNING
START

———————————

PUMPKIN BREAKFAST COOKIES

◇

This is your all-in-one breakfast to go that you can bake, store and eat all week. Freeze these cookies and they'll last even longer! Just take one out of the freezer the night before to defrost and you'll wake up to a sweet breakfast that's ready when you are. And the best part? Not only do they cover all your macronutrient needs – protein, fibre and healthy fats – but they also taste amazing. I love them for an afternoon treat, too!

makes 12 large cookies

Coconut oil to grease baking tray (if not
   using waxed paper)
120g almond butter
120g cooked, puréed pumpkin
85–170g raw honey or maple syrup,
   depending on how sweet you like it
1 large egg
½ teaspoon pure vanilla extract
140g rolled oats
½ teaspoon bicarbonate of soda
30g ground almonds
2 tablespoons chia seeds
2 teaspoons ground cinnamon
50g raisins
40g chopped walnuts (optional)
50g chopped dates or figs (optional)

Preheat the oven to 180°C/gas mark 4. Line a baking tray with waxed paper or grease with coconut oil.

In a large bowl, mix the almond butter, pumpkin purée, honey, egg and vanilla essence.

In a separate medium bowl, mix together the oats, bicarbonate of soda, ground almonds, chia seeds and cinnamon.

Fold the oat mixture into the almond butter mixture.

Fold in the raisins and the walnuts and dates or figs (if using).

Form the mixture into 12 balls and set them 3–5cm apart on the prepared baking tray. Flatten them slightly with your palm. Bake for 15–20 minutes, or until golden brown.

Store in the fridge, loosely covered, for up to 1 week.

tip

REACH FOR NATURAL NUT BUTTER, WITH NO ADDED SUGARS OR OILS, WHENEVER POSSIBLE.

THE BEST BAKED PORRIDGE

◇

Is porridge your favourite breakfast? Then this recipe is for you. Many of my clients love a warm bowl of comforting goodness in the morning, but don't have time to make it everyday. Not only can you make this ahead of time, but this version has more protein, so you'll be ready to face the morning no matter what it looks like. I like to use a bun tin to make cute little muffins that are delicious at room temperature or warmed up in the oven.

serves 6

Oil, for greasing tins

140g rolled oats

1–2 teaspoons ground cinnamon

1 teaspoon baking powder

½ teaspoon sea salt

¼ teaspoon freshly grated nutmeg

2 tablespoons chia seeds

115g pure maple syrup or honey

2 large eggs

3 tablespoons unsalted butter or coconut
   oil, melted

400ml milk of choice

EXTRAS

Apple Cinnamon: 180g diced apple,
   2 teaspoons ground cinnamon

Blackberry Coconut: 115g blackberries, cut
   in half; 40g desiccated coconut

Chai Spice: ½ teaspoon ground cinnamon,
   1 teaspoon each ground ginger and ground
   cardamom, freshly ground black pepper

Preheat the oven to 180°C/gas mark 4. Grease a 20cm square baking dish or tin or a bun tin.

In a large bowl, combine all the ingredients, plus extra ingredients of your choice, and stir until everything is mixed evenly.

Bake for about 40 minutes, if using a baking dish, or about 25 minutes for individual muffins. The baked porridge is done when it turns golden brown and feels firm to the touch.

If you used a baking dish, turn out onto a wire rack to cool, then transfer to a cutting board and cut it into six even squares or slices. If you used a bun tin, transfer the muffins to a wire rack to cool. The baked porridge will keep in the fridge for 5–7 days.

VARIATION
Soak the oats in 120g buttermilk and 475g water for 15–20 minutes before step 2, and omit the 400ml milk.

tip

I LIKE USING SILICONE BUN TINS AND BAKING DISHES
BECAUSE THEY'RE NATURALLY NON-STICK.

$\diamond$

BIBIMBAP BREAKFAST BOWL

If you're looking for something savoury for breakfast instead of smoothies or yogurt, this grain-free bibimbap-style bowl will help switch your sweet morning routine. Plus, this bowl is a perfect vessel for homemade gut-friendly kimchi (see page 147).

---

serves 1

150g cauliflower florets

Coconut oil, for frying

About 100g greens, e.g. kale, baby kale, spinach or rocket

1 teaspoon toasted sesame oil, plus more for serving if wished

1 large egg

About 50g grated carrot

About 50g bean sprouts

1–2 tablespoons kimchi (see page 147) or fermented radishes (see page 144)

1 spring onion, sliced diagonally

Pulse the cauliflower in a food processor until the mixture resembles couscous.

In a medium frying pan, melt the coconut oil over medium heat. Add the cauliflower rice and cook until warmed through, about 3–5 minutes, then transfer it to your bowl.

Add the greens to the frying pan and cook until wilted, 2–4 minutes Drizzle the greens with the toasted sesame oil and place in your bowl.

If necessary, melt a little more coconut oil in the pan, then crack in the egg and fry to your desired doneness.

Add the carrots and bean sprouts to the bowl. Top with the fried egg and garnish with kimchi or fermented radishes, spring onion and more sesame oil, if wished.

tip

YOU CAN SWAP THE CAULIFLOWER RICE FOR ANY GRAIN THAT WORKS FOR YOU (WHITE OR BROWN RICE, QUINOA, AND MORE).

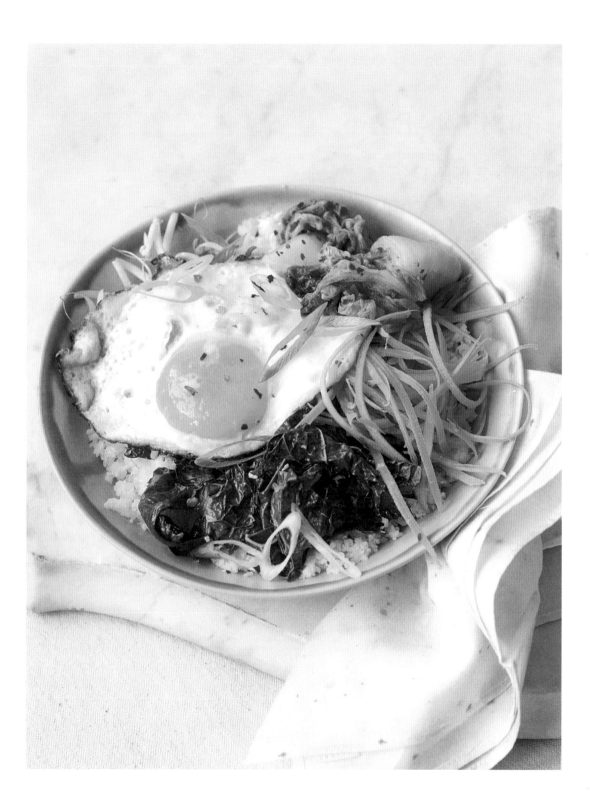

HOMEMADE COCONUT YOGURT

◇

I love yogurt and typically use goats' milk yogurt in my Power Parfait (see page 36), but I know some of my community can't do dairy. This fun little recipe doesn't have complicated steps or require extra kitchen gadgets (except a thermometer). With its good-for-your-gut probiotics and grass-fed gelatin, this yogurt is amazing for healing your gut lining which helps you digest your food properly and assimilate all the good nutrients you're eating.

makes about 1.2 litres

3 x 400ml tins full-fat coconut milk

1 tablespoon grass-fed gelatin

1–2 tablespoons raw honey or pure maple syrup, depending on how sweet you like it

¼ teaspoon yogurt starter (available at your local health foods shop or online)

tip

SINCE THIS YOGURT CONTAINS GELATIN, IT DOESN'T INTEGRATE IN MOST RECIPES AS WELL AS TRADITIONAL DAIRY YOGURT. IF YOU WANT TO MAKE MY POWER PARFAIT WITH IT, I RECOMMEND BLENDING THE PROTEIN POWDER, OATS AND CHIA SEEDS WITH THE YOGURT IN A BLENDER OR FOOD-PROCESSOR. THEN SCOOP THE MIXTURE BACK INTO YOUR CONTAINER AND PLACE IT IN THE FRIDGE TO RE-SET.

In a saucepan, heat the coconut milk over medium heat until it registers 82°C on a kitchen thermometer.

In a small bowl, dissolve the gelatin in a small amount of water. Whisk in a few tablespoons of the hot coconut milk, then pour this mixture into the pan with the coconut milk. Remove from the heat and thoroughly mix in your sweetener of choice.

Cover and leave to cool to 35°–38°C. Transfer half the yogurt mixture to a bowl and stir in the yogurt starter. Add the remaining yogurt mixture and mix well. Pour the yogurt mixture into sterilised 250–500ml preserving jars or other sterilised containers.

Cover and set aside to ferment at 40°–46°C – this can be done by putting the jars in the oven and turning the light on (leave the oven itself off).

Ferment the yogurt for up to 24 hours. Taste the yogurt and see how you like it after 7 hours. When it tastes tangy enough for you, give it a stir and transfer it to the fridge. (Note that the yogurt will not thicken until it has been refrigerated for a few hours.)

Store in the fridge for up to 2 weeks.

◇

GREEN GIRL GRANOLA

If you love my Power Parfaits and want to get creative in the kitchen making your own granola, this is my favourite go-to recipe. Cardamom is the superstar here – this Ayurvedic cooling spice has a unique taste and is great for soothing digestive issues. You can make a huge batch of this crunchy, nutrient-dense medley and store it in jars for weeks. Just keep it in a dry, cool place to extend its shelf life.

serves 8

110g rolled oats

40g flaxseeds

40g hemp seeds

30g pumpkin seeds

40g chia seeds

150g dried fruit (e.g. dates, apricots or figs),
    roughly chopped

2 teaspoons ground cinnamon

1 teaspoon ground cardamom

85g raw honey or pure maple syrup

2 teaspoons pure vanilla extract

3 tablespoons coconut oil or unsalted
    butter, melted

1–2 teaspoons matcha powder (optional;
    this gives the granola a nice green colour)

Preheat the oven to 160°C/gas mark 3.

In a large bowl, combine the oats, seeds, dried fruit, cinnamon and cardamom and mix together.

In a small bowl, stir together the honey or maple syrup, vanilla and coconut oil or butter.

Add the wet mixture to the dry and stir to combine.

Spread the granola in an even layer on a rimmed baking tray and bake for 15–20 minutes, or until golden.

Remove the granola from the oven and leave to cool cool on the tray. Sprinkle the matcha powder, if using, over the granola mixture and toss to combine.

Transfer to jars and store at room temperature in a cool, dry place for up to several weeks.

tip

IF YOUR HONEY CRYSTALLISES IT MEANS YOU'VE GOT THE REAL STUFF! TO RETURN IT TO LIQUID CONSISTENCY, PLACE THE JAR IN A BOWL OF HOT WATER FOR A FEW MINUTES.

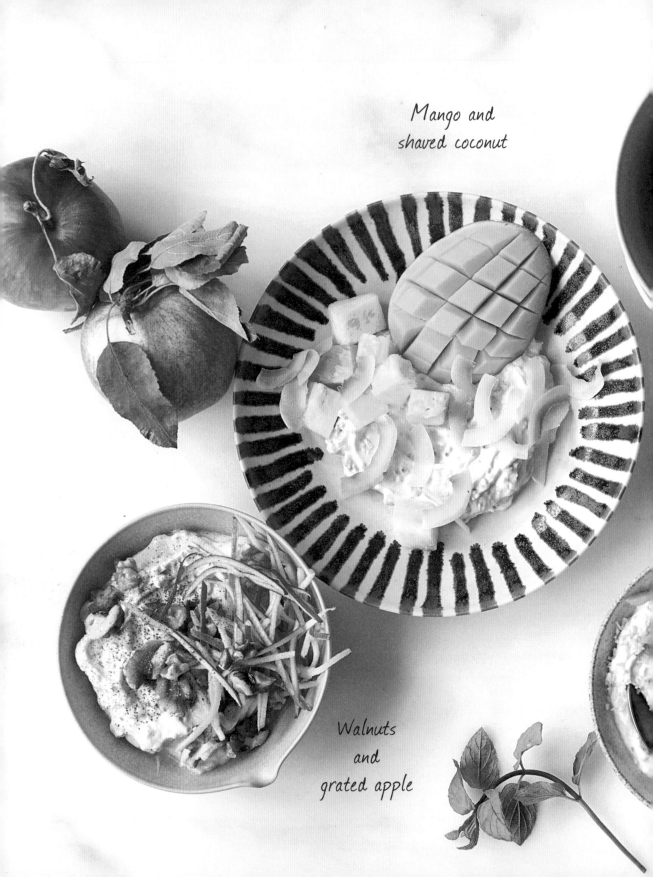

Mango and
shaved coconut

Walnuts
and
grated apple

POWER PARFAIT

FIRST, START WITH THE BASE RECIPE ON PAGE 36. THEN CUSTOMIZE TOPPINGS TO YOUR TASTE. HERE ARE SOME IDEAS TO GET YOU STARTED.

Make It Your Way!

Fresh berry mix and mint

Mashed cooked sweet potato swirl with almonds

Nectarines, fresh figs, and almond slivers

GO-GO
EGG MUFFIN

Not only are these muffins packed with veggies, but the addition of ground almonds makes them feel more substantial than, say, a frittata. Pop a few of them in a tuppaware for a breakfast on-the-go, or enjoy them as a protein-filled snack.

makes about 8 muffins

Oil, for greasing

About 200g grated vegetables (I recommend courgettes, carrots and parsnips)

2 large eggs

2 tablespoons coconut oil, melted

85g ground almonds

¼ teaspoon bicarbonate of soda

¼ teaspoon baking powder

½ teaspoon sea salt

¼ teaspoon freshly ground black pepper

1 tablespoon Italian seasoning

Preheat the oven to 180°C/gas mark 4. Grease 8 cups of a standard bun tin.

In a large bowl, combine the grated vegetables, eggs, coconut oil, ground almonds, bicarbonate of soda, baking powder, salt, pepper and Italian seasoning. Mix until combined.

Pour the batter into the prepared cups of the bun tin and bake for 20–25 minutes, or until golden brown.

Store in an airtight container in the fridge for up to 4 days.

BLUEBERRY CHIA MUFFIN

When I was growing up in Long Island, I used to go to the mall for giant, white-flour-laden blueberry muffins the size of my head. I still love real muffins, so I wanted to come up with a healthy version that's just as yummy without the sugar crash. Make a batch of these in advance for quick breakfasts and treats throughout the week. They also freeze beautifully.

makes 12 muffins

80g coconut oil, melted and cooled, plus
   more for greasing
60ml milk of choice
2 large eggs
375g thick, Greek-style yogurt
1 teaspoon pure vanilla extract
240g gluten-free flour
75g coconut sugar
2 teaspoons baking powder
Pinch of sea salt
40g chia seeds
¼ teaspoon ground cinnamon
200g fresh blueberries

Preheat the oven to 160°C/gas mark 3. Grease a standard bun tin.

In a large bowl, stir together the coconut oil, milk, eggs, yogurt and vanilla.

In a medium bowl, mix together the flour, coconut sugar, baking powder, salt, chia seeds and cinnamon.

Add the flour mixture to the coconut oil mixture in three additions, mixing well after each.

Fold the blueberries into the batter and then divide the batter evenly among the cups of the prepared bun tin.

Bake for 25–35 minutes, or until a skewer inserted into the middle of a muffin comes out clean. Leave to cool in the tin on a wire rack. Store in the fridge, loosely covered, for up to 1 week.

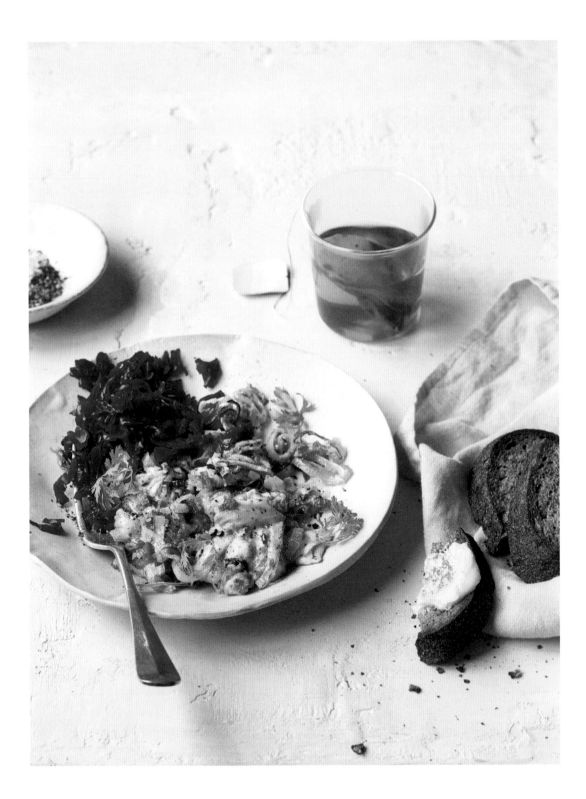

◇

IMMUNITY SCRAMBLE

This stellar scrambled-egg recipe was developed by my cooking assistant, Gaby, and is packed with gut-nourishing, immune-boosting ingredients such as ginger, turmeric and leeks. Fresh turmeric can turn your hands and clothes (and countertops!) a vibrant yellow colour, so if you're worried about staining, I recommend wearing gloves and an apron, and using a little caution while grating the root. This delightful dish is definitely worth the effort, though!

---

serves 2

1½ teaspoons coconut oil or grass-fed butter

60g leek, chopped

1cm piece of ginger, peeled and grated

5mm piece of turmeric, peeled and grated

4 large eggs, beaten

Sea salt and freshly ground black pepper

In a medium frying pan, melt the coconut oil or butter over medium heat. Add the leek and cook, stirring, until caramelised, 5–6 minutes.

Add the ginger and turmeric and cook, stirring, for a minute more, until fragrant.

Add the eggs, season with salt and pepper and cook, stirring to scramble the eggs, until they are cooked to the consistency of your liking.

tip

FOR EXTRA-CREAMY EGGS, BRING A SMALL POT OF WATER TO A BOIL WHILE YOU'RE COOKING THE LEEKS IN STEP 1. WHEN YOU'RE READY TO ADD THE EGGS IN STEP 3, REMOVE THE PAN FROM THE HEAT AND SET IT OVER THE POT OF BOILING WATER – THE STEAM FROM THE WATER HEATS THE PAN AND COOKS THE EGGS SLOWLY, AND THEY COME OUT SUPER FLUFFY!

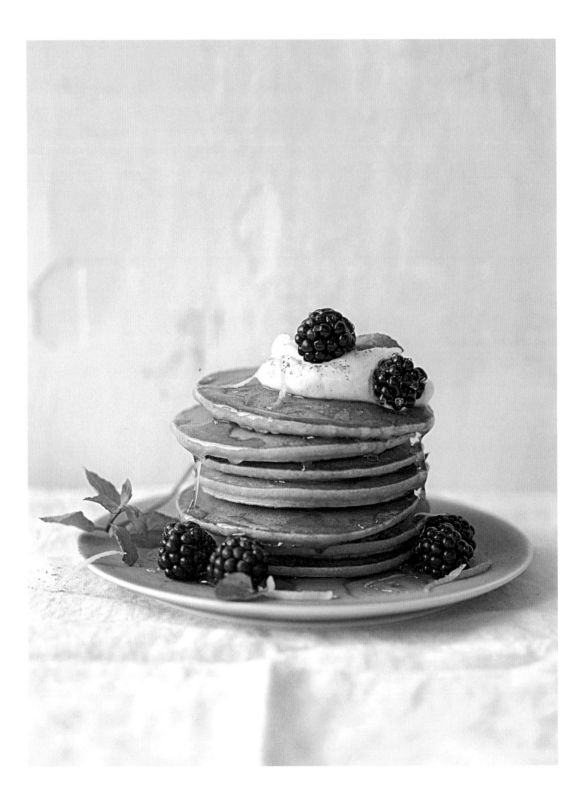

◇

ACTIVATED
CORN CAKES

Eating less gluten in our day-to-day lives doesn't mean we can't satisfy those carb-food cravings – they just need an upgrade! These little pancakes are a perfect addition to your Sunday batch cooking and are so versatile. Heat them up in the oven and top with avocado, egg and sauerkraut for a quick lunch – just don't forget your greens on the side – or, if you're hungry at 4 o'clock, you topping one with almond butter for a snack.

---

serves 4–6

250g fine cornmeal

120g oat flour

350ml buttermilk

2 large eggs

1 tablespoon pure vanilla extract

Pinch of sea salt

½ teaspoon baking powder

85g raw honey

Squeeze of fresh lemon juice

1 tablespoon coconut oil, for frying

Toppings of your choice, sweet or savoury

In a medium bowl, whisk together the cornmeal, oat flour, buttermilk and 120ml water and leave to stand for 10 minutes.

In a large bowl, combine the eggs, vanilla, salt, baking powder, honey and lemon juice.

Add the flour mixture to the egg mixture and mix to combine.

In a large frying pan, melt the coconut oil over medium–low heat. Spoon 4 tablespoons of the batter into the pan. Flip the pancake when bubbles appear on the surface and cook on the other side until golden brown.

Go sweet and serve with your favourite pancake toppings, or experiment with something savoury.

tip

YOU CAN MAKE THE BATTER AND STORE IT IN THE FRIDGE FOR UP TO 3 DAYS TO USE FOR FRESH PANCAKES EVERY MORNING!

◇

GOLDEN MILK SMOOTHIE

This smoothie combines healing spices with lucuma, a nutrient-dense, low-glycaemic sweetener made from a Peruvian fruit. Lucuma is also rich in prebiotic fibre (which feeds those good probiotics in your gut).

serves 1

150g frozen courgette, steamed

240ml non-dairy milk (I recommend coconut or cashew for this recipe)

1½ teaspoons chia seeds

1 teaspoon ground turmeric

1cm piece of ginger, peeled

1 teaspoon pure vanilla extract

2 teaspoons ground cinnamon

1 tablespoon lucuma powder (optional)

Pinch of freshly ground black pepper

20g rolled oats

Combine all the ingredients in a high-speed blender and blend until smooth.

BLUEBERRY PIE SMOOTHIE

If banana smoothies give you a sugar high and upset your tummy, frozen steamed cauliflower is your new best friend. This secret, tasteless ingredient gives you all the creaminess with none of the sugar that bananas contain.

serves 1

180g frozen cauliflower, steamed

About 2–4 tablespoons collagen

75g frozen blueberries

350ml non-dairy milk (I recommend almond or flax for this recipe)

½ teaspoon ground cinnamon

½ teaspoon pure vanilla extract

1 teaspoon chia seeds

1 teaspoon nut butter

1 or 2 drops of liquid stevia (optional)

Combine all the ingredients except the stevia in a high-speed blender and blend until smooth. Taste and add a drop or two of stevia, if wished, and blend to incorporate before serving.

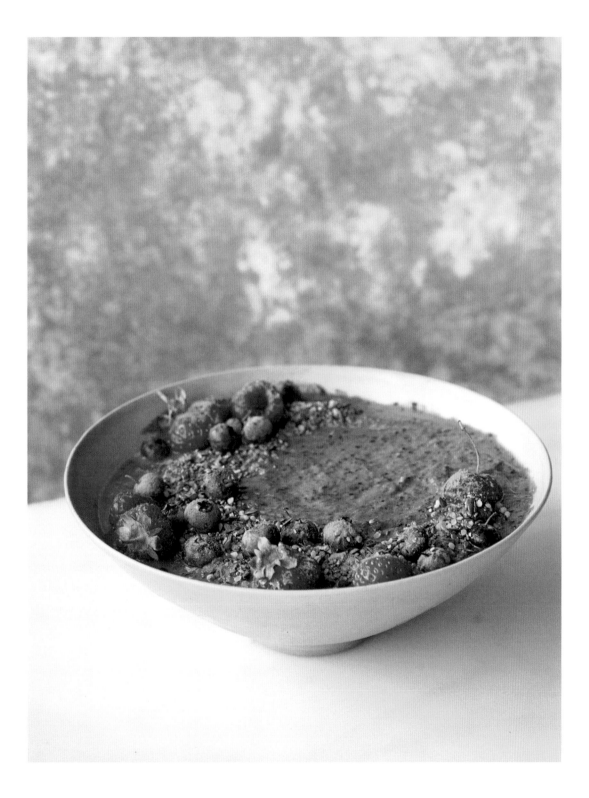

◊

NEW FAVE SMOOTHIE

This smoothie is a unusual way to use up leftover sweet potatoes, providing an easy vehicle to incorporate more of this root veggie into your diet. Don't have cooked sweet potato to hand? Try substituting pumpkin!

serves 1

100g cooked and
   mashed sweet potato
½ large banana,
   peeled and frozen
240ml non-dairy milk
   (I recommend almond
   or coconut for this
   recipe)
25g raw walnut halves
1cm piece of ginger,
   peeled

Pinch of ground
   cinnamon, plus
   extra for sprinkling
   (optional)
½ teaspoon maca
   powder (optional)
1 Medjool date, pitted
   (optional)
3 ice cubes

Combine all the ingredients in a high-speed blender and blend until smooth. Garnish with an additional sprinkle of cinnamon, if wished.

◊

'PEAS, PLEASE' SMOOTHIE

This smoothie might sound a little weird, but it's actually amazingly refreshing and flavourful. Avocado makes it creamy, peas provide extra fibre, banana sweetens it up, and all that spinach will make you feel like a green goddess!

serves 1

Flesh of ¼ large or
   ½ small avocado
75g frozen peas
1 banana, peeled and
   frozen
350ml non-dairy milk
   (I recommend almond
   or coconut for this
   recipe)
Generous handful of
   baby spinach

1–2 scoops vanilla
   protein powder
   (about 2–4
   tablespoons)
1 teaspoon pure vanilla
   extract
1 teaspoon
   tocotrienols
3 ice cubes

Combine all the ingredients in a high-speed blender and blend until smooth.

◇

BREAKFAST SALAD

Have you ever heard the saying 'How you do one thing is how you do everything'? Well, I'd like to take it up a notch and say 'How you do BREAKFAST is how you do everything'! Starting your day on a healthy note has a domino effect on the rest of your day. When you start with a nutrient-dense meal, you're way more likely to choose healthy food options all day long.

serves 1

Coconut oil, for frying

1 or 2 large eggs

About 100g greens, e.g. rocket, baby kale or baby spinach

Good-quality extra-virgin olive oil

70g cubed roasted or steamed sweet potato, at room temperature or warm

1 or 2 tablespoons sauerkraut, for serving, plus a drizzle of the fermentation juice

Sliced or diced flesh of ¼ avocado

Gomasio (see Note), for garnish (optional)

Sea salt and freshly ground black pepper

In a small frying pan, melt enough coconut oil over medium heat to coat the bottom of the pan.

Crack the egg(s) into the frying pan and cook to your liking.

Put the greens in a bowl and drizzle lightly with olive oil. Toss to coat the leaves. Top with the sweet potato, sauerkraut, avocado and egg(s). Drizzle with a little of the sauerkraut juice.

Sprinkle with gomasio, if wished, and season with salt and pepper.

tip

YOU CAN ALSO LIGHTLY STEAM THE GREENS FOR A WARMER VARIATION.

note

FOR A WARMER VARIATION, LIGHTLY STEAM THE GREENS. GOMASIO IS A JAPANESE CONDIMENT MADE OF SESAME SEEDS AND SALT; IT'S DELICIOUS HERE, AS WELL AS ON SOUPS AND PLAIN-COOKED PROTEINS AND GRAINS.

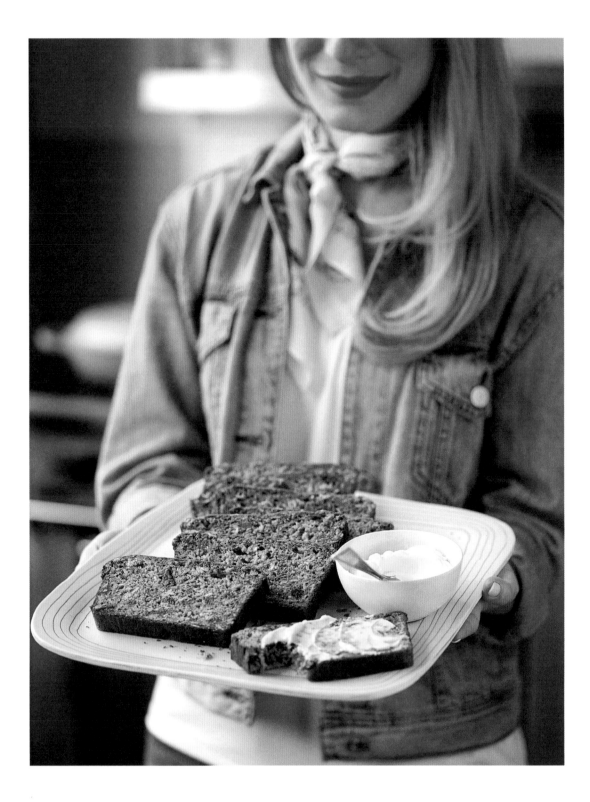

◇

SUPERWOMAN
BREAD

When my sister-in-law had a baby, I made her this bread to have on hand during her marathon nursing sessions, and froze it in slices that were easy to reheat. This bread is very good for women's hormonal health, with the addition of ground flaxseed and goji berries. There's no kneading or complex fermentation process involved here, but it comes out like a real loaf of bread.

makes 1 loaf

Oil, for greasing

2 tablespoons ground flaxseed

210g gluten-free flour

90g rolled oats

½ teaspoon sea salt

1 teaspoon bicarbonate of soda

½ teaspoon ground cinnamon

30g goji berries

2 tablespoons chia seeds

2 tablespoons hemp seeds

50g dried apricots, chopped

115g unsalted butter,
  at room temperature

3 large eggs

150g coconut sugar or date sugar

300g natural yogurt

2 tablespoons milk of choice

1 teaspoon pure vanilla extract

2 tablespoons orange zest

Preheat the oven to 180°C/gas mark 4. Grease a standard 23 x 13cm loaf tin.

In a large bowl, mix together the ground flaxseed, flour, oats, salt, bicarbonate of soda, cinnamon, goji berries, chia and hemp seeds and apricots.

In a separate large bowl, mix the butter, eggs, coconut sugar, yogurt, milk, vanilla and orange zest.

Slowly add the flour mixture to the butter mixture and mix thoroughly to combine.

Pour the batter into the prepared loaf tin and bake for 1 hour, or until a skewer inserted into the center comes out clean.

Remove the loaf from the tin and leave to cool on a wire rack. Wrapped in foil or a clean tea-towel, it will keep for a couple of days, or you can slice and freeze it to enjoy later.

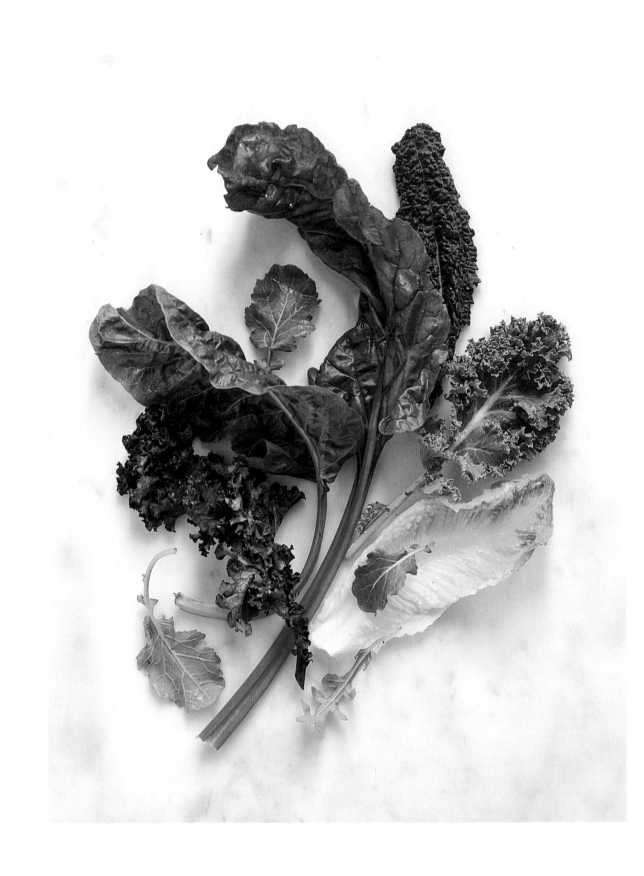

SALADS
AND SOUPS

◇

BLUEBERRY AND ROCKET SALAD

My secret to the best salads ever? Add blueberries. Seriously, I could eat this salad every day of the summer and not get sick of it – it's that good! Also, I find that when I add some naturally sweet fruits and veggies to my meals, I'm much less likely to crave that 'something sweet' afterwards.

---

serves 1

90–180g cooked quinoa

150g rocket

2 carrots, peeled into ribbons or grated

Juice of 1 lemon

2 tablespoons extra-virgin olive oil

Sea salt and freshly ground black pepper

50g fresh blueberries

40g roasted unsalted hazelnuts, sliced, or
   flaked almonds

25g goats' cheese, crumbled (optional)

HOMEMADE HONEY MUSTARD

120g plain yogurt
   (thick Greek-style works best)

3 tablespoons Dijon mustard

2 tablespoons raw honey

3 tablespoons lemon juice

60ml extra-virgin olive oil

Sea salt and black pepper to taste

In a large bowl, combine the quinoa, rocket and carrots.

Dress with the lemon juice and olive oil and season with salt and pepper.

Top with the blueberries and nuts and the crumbled goats' cheese, if using.

Alternatively, you can dress the salad with the Homemade Honey Mustard: Combine the yogurt, mustard, honey, and lemon juice in a medium bowl. Slowly add the oil, whisking constantly until well blended. Add the salt and pepper. You won't need all of it to dress this salad; save the rest in an airtight container in the fridge, where it will keep for up to one week.

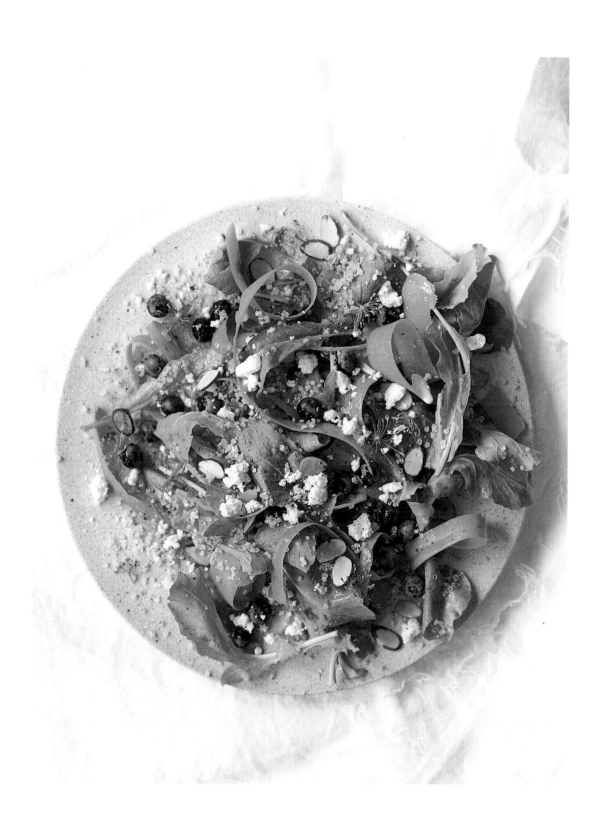

◇

SPRING GREEN SALAD WRAPS

There's something about the combination of spring greens and naturally salty nori sheets that make these wraps oh-so craveable. These wraps meet the Good Gut Rule of Five, making them the perfect alternative to a typical salad or bowl meal. Plus, they're fun to eat! Feel free to use the recipe below as a guideline to experiment with your wrap ingredients!

serves 1

2 spring green leaves, stem removed

2–3 sheets of nori

Optional: hummus, beetroot hummus, tahini
   or other spread of choice

Smoked salmon or smoked turkey breast

About 80g roasted veggies (carrots and
   sweet potatoes are my favourites here)

Sliced flesh of ½ avocado

½ apple, sliced (optional)

Sauerkraut

Fresh herbs

Lay the spring green leaves on a flat surface and place a nori sheet on top of each leaf. If you're using a spread like hummus, spread it over half of each sheet.

Layer the smoked salmon or turkey, roasted veggies, avocado, apple slices if using, sauerkraut and herbs on top, making sure you keep the toppings on just half of the nori sheet so you can roll it up.

Roll up like you would a burrito, folding in the bottom to keep all your toppings in.

Enjoy immediately or wrap up in foil for a quick meal on the go!

CLEANSING FENNEL SALAD

Fennel is a celery-like vegetable with an interesting liquorice flavour, and it's one of the ultimate Go with Your Gut weight-loss foods. It's exceptionally high in fibre, which helps move food through your digestive tract. It's also been used for centuries after meals to prevent stomach upset. This simple salad is one of my favourite ways to highlight this underused veggie. If you eat dairy, try topping the salad with a few thin slices of Parmesan.

serves 4

1 fennel bulb, thinly sliced, 1 tablespoon
   fronds chopped and reserved for garnish
   if wished

2 celery stalks, thinly sliced

1 kohlrabi, peeled and cut into matchsticks
   (optional)

Juice of ½ lemon

2 tablespoons extra-virgin olive oil

Sea salt and freshly ground black pepper

Toasted pine nuts, flaked almonds or
   pumpkin seeds, to garnish (optional)

In a large bowl, combine the sliced fennel, celery and kohlrabi, if using.

Sprinkle over the lemon juice and olive oil and season with salt and pepper to taste. Toss to combine.

Garnish with the reserved fennel fronds and nuts or pumpkin seeds, if using, before serving.

◇

SMOKED TROUT AND LENTIL SALAD

Inspired by one of my favourite restaurants in New York City, Café Gitane, this salad is exactly the sort of thing you want to be eating while sitting on a café terrace and sipping rosé. The lentils fill you up, keep you energised and ensure your digestion is moving along, while smoked trout is full of omegas that are great for healthy skin. If you prefer, you can substitute sardines or smoked mussels.

serves 4

200g beluga lentils

1 avocado

70g cherry tomatoes, halved

50g goats' cheese, crumbled

40g walnuts, coarsely chopped

50g raisins or dried cranberries

80g rocket

2 smoked trout fillets, skins removed if
 possible, cut into pieces

ROASTED SHALLOT VINAIGRETTE

2 medium shallots, halved

3 garlic cloves

120ml extra virgin olive oil, plus extra for
 drizzling

60ml apple cider vinegar

Small handful of fresh flat-leaf parsley

1 teaspoon Dijon mustard

½ teaspoon sea salt

Pinch of freshly ground black pepper

Put the lentils and 500ml of water in a pan over medium high heat and bring to the boil. Cover the pan, reduce the heat and simmer for about 20–30 minutes, or until the lentils are tender. Drain any excess water.

Make the vinaigrette. Preheat the oven to 200°C/ gas mark 6. Place the shallots and garlic on a baking tray and drizzle with olive oil. Roast until just lightly browned, about 15 minutes. Leave to cool slightly.

Transfer the garlic and shallots to a blender. Add the olive oil, vinegar, parsley, mustard, salt and pepper and blend until smooth. Add a little more olive oil to thin it out, if needed.

Dice the flesh of the avocado and put in a large bowl, together with the lentils, tomatoes, goats' cheese, walnuts and raisins or cranberries. Pour over vinaigrette to taste and toss gently to combine.

Divide the rocket among four plates and top with a generous scoop of the lentil salad and the pieces of smoked trout.

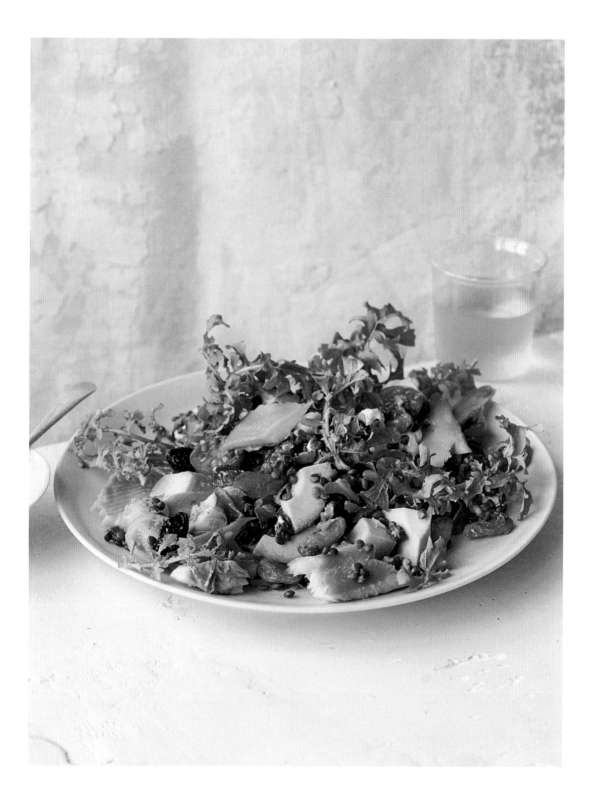

◇

'CHEESY' BROCCOLI SOUP

This dairy-free soup tastes just as good (if not better) than the classic and won't leave you feeling bloated. The secret ingredient is nutritional yeast, a product made from deactivated yeast, which is rich in B vitamins. It has a nutty, tangy flavour, which is why it's often used as a cheese substitute in vegan and paleo recipes. Most of these ingredients are pantry staples.

serves 6

1 tablespoon butter or ghee

1 small onion, chopped

Sea salt and freshly ground black pepper

2 garlic cloves, crushed

450g broccoli florets (from about 2 heads), chopped

25g nutritional yeast

Juice of ½ lemon (about 2 tablespoons)

1 small bunch of fresh parsley, chopped

1 x 400ml tin coconut milk (optional)

In a large saucepan, melt the butter over medium heat. Add the onion, season with salt and pepper and cook, stirring, for 5–7 minutes.

Add the garlic and cook, stirring, for a few minutes more, until fragrant.

Add 1 litre of water and bring to the boil. Add the broccoli and cook until bright green, about 3–4 minutes.

Remove the pan from the heat and carefully transfer the soup to a blender or food-processor (you may need to do this in batches). Add the nutritional yeast, lemon juice and parsley. If you like the taste and creaminess of coconut milk, add that too.

Blend until smooth (be careful when blending hot liquids). Alternatively, blend the soup directly in the pot using a stick blender.

Serve immediately or store in an airtight container in the fridge for up to 5 days.

UMAMI MUSHROOM SOUP

Mushrooms are totally trending right now. There's a reason mushrooms are so popular – they're packed with key minerals like selenium, copper, potassium and iron. Mushrooms also especially good if you don't eat much meat – they're rich in 'umami' flavour, which is often what you're really looking for when you crave meat.

serves 3–4

2 tablespoons dried mushrooms (shiitake, morel, chanterelle)

4 tablespoons unsalted butter or ghee

2 leeks, thinly sliced and well washed

Sea salt

4 garlic cloves, thinly sliced

About 400g fresh mushrooms (choose a mix of cremini, oyster, chanterelle, button and portobello), chopped

Freshly ground black pepper

240ml bone broth or vegetable stock

2 tablespoons chopped fresh sage

1 tablespoon fresh thyme leaves (or 1 teaspoon dried)

Dash of champagne or red wine vinegar

Put the dried mushrooms in a small bowl and cover with boiling water. Leave to soak for 20 minutes to rehydrate. Scoop out the mushrooms and set aside. Line a fine-mesh sieve with a coffee filter and strain the soaking liquid. Set aside.

In a large saucepan, melt the butter over medium heat. Add the leeks and a pinch of salt and cook, stirring, for 5 minutes. Add the garlic and cook, stirring, until fragrant.

Add the fresh mushrooms and season with salt and pepper, then add the rehydrated dried mushrooms and their soaking water, the bone broth or stock and 240ml water and bring to the boil.

Reduce the heat to maintain a simmer. Add the sage and thyme, cover and cook for 15–20 minutes.

If wished, use up to 60ml more water to thin the soup to your liking. Add a splash of vinegar. Serve the soup as is, blend it or blend half and mix it back in.

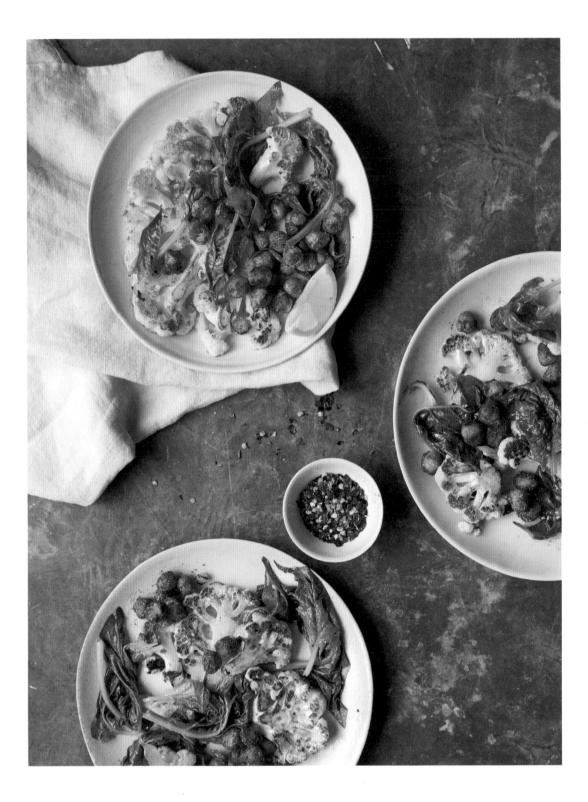

WARM CAULIFLOWER SALAD

◇

From an Ayurvedic perspective, raw foods are cold, dry, light and rough. Consuming too much of these foods can strain our digestion, which can lead to poor absorption of nutrients, bloating and other discomfort. Enter the warm salad! I created this salad for those who have trouble digesting raw greens, but ended up loving it so much that it's now become a winter lunchtime classic. Warming a salad is also a great way to make a plate of veggies feel more like a full meal.

serves 4

SPICED CHICKPEAS

2 tablespoons olive or avocado oil

1 x 400g tin chickpeas, drained and rinsed

½ teaspoon ground cumin

¼ teaspoon paprika

¼ teaspoon crushed chillies

Sea salt and freshly ground black pepper

SALAD

2 tablespoons olive or avocado oil

½ cauliflower, sliced

150g fresh spinach

Lemon wedges, for serving

To make the spiced chickpeas, in a large frying pan, heat the oil over medium heat. Add the chickpeas, cumin, paprika, crushed chillies and salt and black pepper to taste. Cook the chickpeas, stirring occasionally, until crisp, 12–15 minutes. Transfer to a plate.

In the same pan, heat the remaining 2 tablespoons of oil. Add the cauliflower and cook, stirring, until browned on both sides.

Add the spinach, return the chickpeas to the pan and cook, stirring, until the spinach is slightly wilted.

Serve with lemon wedges for squeezing over the top.

◇

GRILLED SALAD

Grilling is an underused technique when it comes to preparing salad greens. Charring your romaine a little gives an amazing smoky, rich flavour. This is a great side dish for summer barbecues and you can even cook your romaine in a griddle pan for a delicious dish at any time of year.

---

serves 4

4 teaspoons chopped fresh herbs, e.g. rosemary, thyme, tarragon and oregano

60ml extra-virgin olive oil

1 tablespoon apple cider vinegar

¼ teaspoon sea salt, plus more as needed

Pinch of freshly ground black pepper

3 heads of cos lettuce, halved lengthways through the core

3 heads of red or white chicory, halved lengthways through the core

Prepare a grill for high, direct heat, or heat a cast-iron frying pan or griddle pan on the hob over high heat.

In a medium bowl, whisk together the herbs, olive oil, vinegar, salt and pepper.

Brush the cos and chicory halves all over with the vinaigrette.

Grill the cos and chicory until lightly browned on all sides, 4–5 minutes, turning halfway through.

Serve immediately, either whole or chopped and tossed in a bowl as a salad.

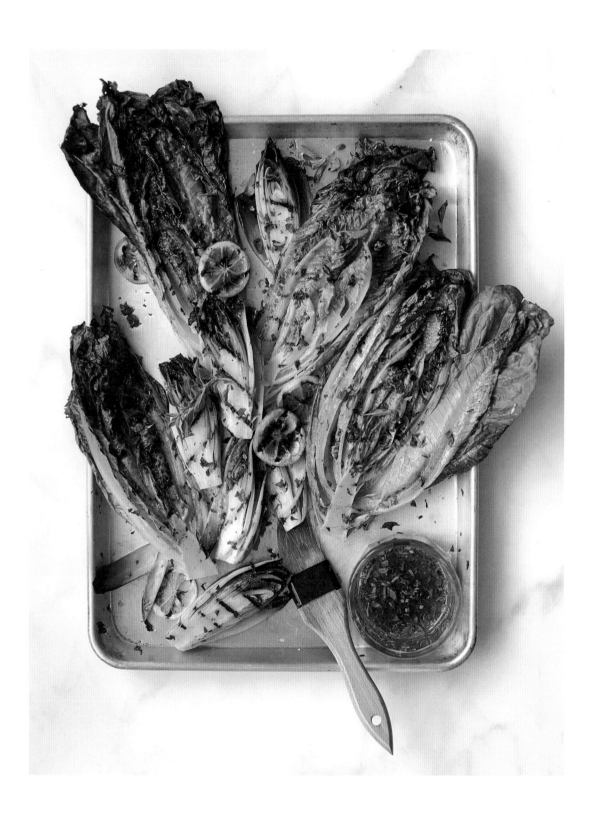

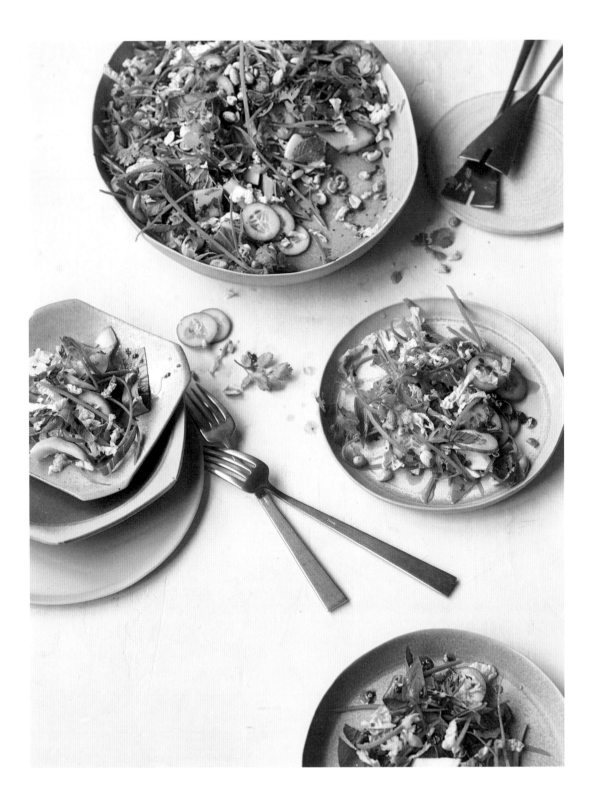

◇

CRUNCHITY VIETNAMESE SALAD

The unusual star ingredient of this salad is pak choi. Pak choi is chock-full of vitamins (A, C, and K) and minerals (calcium, magnesium, potassium, manganese and iron), and I'm always trying to eat more of this super veggie. This salad is crisp and flavourful, bursting with fresh herbs and lime. Pair it with grilled prawns, tofu or fish for a light dinner. You can also add rice or quinoa for a heartier meal.

---

serves about 8

1 large pak choi, thinly sliced

½ small head of Chinese leaf, shredded

1 carrot, thinly sliced

1 cucumber, peeled and thinly sliced (if you're using a smaller, Persian-style cucumber, you can leave the skin on)

½ bunch of coriander, chopped

3 tablespoons chopped fresh mint leaves

3 spring onions, thinly sliced

35g peanuts, crushed, for garnish (optional)

DRESSING

Juice of 3 limes

1 tablespoon toasted sesame oil

1½ tablespoons rice vinegar

3 tablespoons tamari or coconut aminos

1–2 teaspoons crushed chillies

Sea salt and freshly ground black pepper

Make the dressing. In small bowl, whisk together the lime juice, sesame oil, vinegar, tamari, crushed chillies and salt and black pepper to taste.

In a large salad bowl, combine the pak choi, Chinese leaf, carrot, cucumber, coriander, mint and spring onions and toss to combine.

Add the dressing and toss gently to coat the salad. Garnish with the peanuts, if wished, and serve.

tip

HAVE TROUBLE DIGESTING RAW VEGGIES? YOU CAN TOSS THIS SALAD IN A FRYING PAN FOR A FEW MINUTES WITH THE DRESSING – IT TASTES GREAT EITHER WAY!

◊

HEALING GREENS SOUP

This soup is like rehab for your gut and waistline, which is why it's one of the recipes I use in my Good Gut Reset (see pages 38–47). Loaded with good-for-you (and naturally slimming) ingredients plus tons of dark leafy greens, this soup will leave you feeling deeply nourished. You can sip it between meals as a snack or have a bowl with a poached egg for a more complete reset-style meal.

serves 2–4

2–4 garlic cloves, crushed

2–3cm piece of ginger, peeled and grated

2 bunches of dark leafy greens, e.g.
*   spinach, watercress, kale, mustard greens*
*   and/or spring greens, chopped*

2–3 spring onions, chopped (optional)

1 yellow onion, chopped

3 tablespoons organic miso paste

Sea salt and freshly ground black pepper

Sprinkle of cayenne pepper

Juice of ½ lemon (about 2 tablespoons)

Fresh herbs, to garnish (optional)

In a medium to large saucepan, combine the garlic, ginger and 700ml water and bring to the boil.

Add the greens and reduce the heat to maintain a simmer.

Add the spring onions (if using) and onion and cook for 1–2 minutes, until the greens are tender. You may need to add additional liquid to generously cover the vegetables. Remove the soup from the heat.

In a small bowl, combine the miso paste with a small amount of the soup broth. Combine thoroughly with a fork and then add the miso mixture to the pot (do not return the pot to the heat).

Season with sea salt, freshly ground black pepper, cayenne pepper and lemon juice to taste. Serve as is, or blend the soup directly in the pot using a stick blender until smooth. Garnish with some chopped fresh herbs, if you wish.

◇

SPICED CARROT SOUP

Blended veggie soups are one of my top gut-friendly, weight-loss foods and also among my favourite healthy comfort foods in general. Warm soups are both super satisfying and easy on your belly. This recipe highlights some of my favourite naturally sweet root vegetables which can help curb sugar cravings.

serves 4–6

3 tablespoons olive or coconut oil

1 large onion, quartered

½ teaspoon sea salt, plus more for seasoning

2 garlic cloves, crushed

2 tablespoons grated fresh turmeric or 1½ teaspoons ground

1 tablespoon grated fresh ginger or 1 teaspoon ground

Freshly ground black pepper

8–10 carrots, diced

3 parsnips, peeled and diced

¼ teaspoon ground cinnamon

475ml bone broth or stock of your choice

OPTIONAL GARNISHES

Chopped hazelnuts, toasted

Spiced Chickpeas (see page 107)

Fresh thyme leaves

In a medium to large saucepan, heat 2 tablespoons of the oil over medium heat. Add the onion, season with a little salt and pepper and cook, stirring, until translucent, about 7 minutes

Add the remaining 1 tablespoon oil, the garlic, turmeric and ginger and reduce the heat to low. Season with pepper and cook until the garlic is lightly browned.

Add the carrots, parsnips, cinnamon and salt. Add the stock and 475ml water and bring to the boil. Reduce the heat to maintain a simmer and cook for 20 minutes.

Blend the soup directly in the pot using a stick blender until smooth (or transfer to a regular blender and purée until smooth. Be careful when blending hot liquids).

Ladle or pour into bowls and top with toasted hazelnuts, spiced chickpeas and/or fresh thyme, if you wish.

◇

NOT-YOUR-GRANDMA'S BORSCHT

My husband wouldn't go near borscht, until he tried this. I'm of Eastern European descent and grew up on the stuff (and love it!), but I understand that not everyone feels the same. It's an acquired taste. This version is more like a veggie soup with tons of beets and lentils, but it has that sour-savoury thing going on that's so irresistible with classic borscht. Added bonus: Beets are gut and hormone-balancing.

---

serves 6–8

60ml avocado or olive oil

½ onion, diced

2 or 3 garlic cloves, crushed

2 celery stalks, diced

3 or 4 large beetroot (about 750g), peeled and diced

2 potatoes, peeled and diced

½ head of red cabbage, shredded

Leaves from 4 sprigs of thyme

4 bay leaves

1 teaspoon caraway seeds

100g lentils (black, brown or green)

A large handful of chopped fresh dill

Juice of 1 lemon (about 4 tablespoons)

Sea salt and freshly ground black pepper to taste

In a large saucepan, heat the oil over medium heat. Add the onion, garlic and celery and season generously with salt and pepper. Cook for 5–7 minutes, stirring occasionally.

Add the beetroot, potatoes and cabbage, season with salt and pepper again and cook, stirring, for a further 5–7 minutes.

Add the thyme, bay leaves, caraway seeds and lentils and pour in enough water to cover (about 1.5–2 litres). Bring to the boil, then reduce the heat to maintain a simmer, cover and cook for about 1 hour, or until the lentils are tender and the potatoes and beetroot are easily pierced with a fork. Taste and add more salt and pepper if needed.

Stir in the chopped dill and lemon juice and serve when ready!

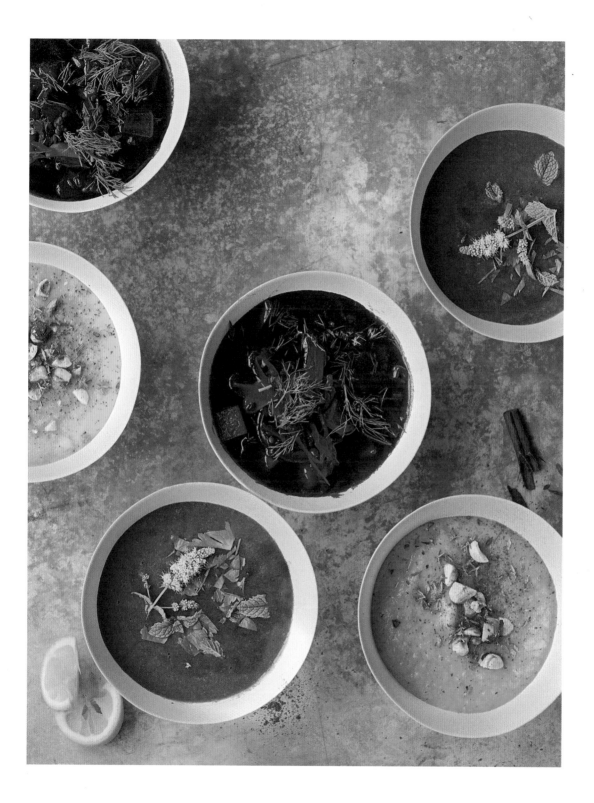

◇

PHO BONE BROTH

This is a fun spin on bone broth, the soup that helps heal your gut lining. Your gut lining works as a barrier between your digestive tract and the rest of your body. If the lining is compromised by poor food choices, stress or environmental toxins, bad bacteria and undigested food may leak from your gut into your body and cause inflammation. Bone broth is my secret weapon, and this Pho version is extra delicious.

makes about 2 litres

2 marrow bones, cut in half lengthways (ask
   your butcher to do this for you)
Sea salt
2 lemongrass stalks
1 cinnamon stick
1 tablespoon coriander seeds
1 tablespoon fennel seeds
1 green cardamom pod
2–3cm piece of ginger, peeled and sliced
2 spring onions, cut into large pieces, plus
   extra sliced spring onion to garnish
Sliced Thai red chillies, to garnish (optional)

tip

LOOKING FOR SOME BASIC BONE
BROTH RECIPES? HEAD TO
ROBYNYOUKILIS.COM/BOOKS!

Preheat the oven to 200°C/gas mark 6. Place the bones on a baking tray, cut side up and sprinkle with salt. Bake for 15 minutes, until the marrow is bubbling. Scoop out the marrow and reserve it for later use (it's great on toast). Put the bones in a large saucepan.

Peel away the tough outer layers of the lemongrass stalks to reveal the pale inner cores and trim the bottoms using a sharp knife. Crush the stems using the flat side of a knife to release the flavour.

Add the crushed lemongrass to the pan with the cinnamon stick, coriander and fennel seeds, cardamom, ginger, spring onion and 2.4 litres of water. Bring to the boil.

Reduce the heat to maintain a simmer, cover and cook for at least 4 hours and up to 8 hours. Strain the broth and discard the bones and veggies.

Ladle some broth into a bowl or mug and garnish with spring onions and/or Thai chillies when you're ready to drink! Let the remaining broth cool to room temperature then store in airtight containers the fridge for up to 5 days or in the freezer for up to 1 year.

HEARTY WINTER STEW

◇

This stew is the ideal all-in-one cold-weather meal. Spring greens are full of iron, protein and fibre, as well as a number of vitamins and minerals. You can use veggie, chicken, turkey or pork sausages in this recipe – they all turn out yummy!

serves about 6

450g any kind of sausage, removed from casing and crumbled or sliced into small bite-sized pieces

Olive oil or ghee for cooking, if needed

1 onion, diced

2 celery stalks, diced

2 carrots, diced

2 garlic cloves, crushed

Sea salt and freshly ground black pepper

2 x 400g tins chopped tomatoes

1 tablespoon tomato purée

1 bunch of spring greens or any kale variety, stems discarded, leaves thinly sliced

In a large saucepan, brown the sausage over medium heat, about 7–8 minutes, then remove and set aside on a plate.

If your pan is dry after cooking the sausage, add 1–2 tablespoons of oil or ghee. Add the onion, celery, carrots and garlic to the pan, season with salt and pepper and cook, stirring, until soft, 8–10 minutes.

Return the sausage and any juices from the plate to the pan. Add the tomatoes and tomato purée and season with a little more salt.

Add 240–470ml water and bring to a simmer. Cover and simmer for 20 minutes.

Add the spring greens and cook until wilted, about 5 minutes more. Serve and enjoy.

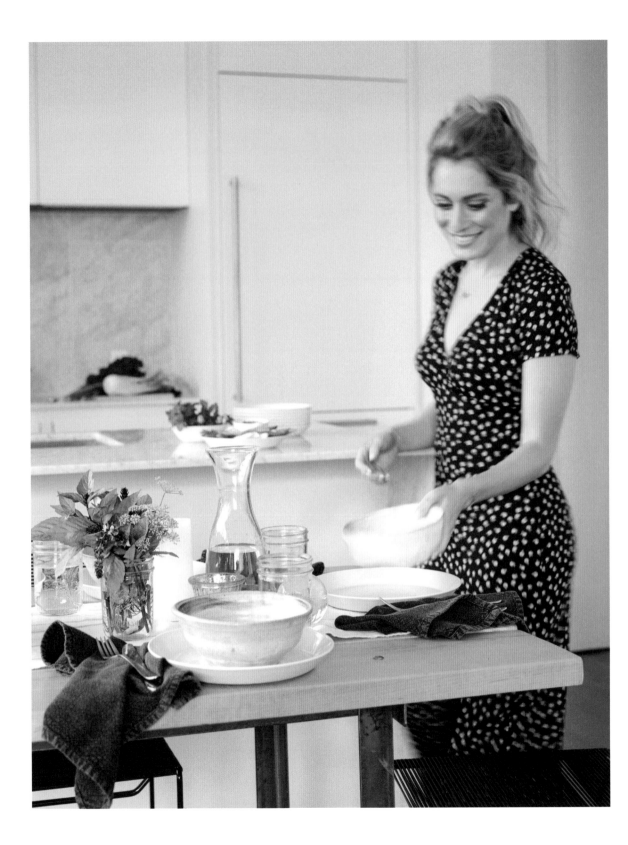

◇

THE
MAIN EVENT

CLASSIC LAMB TAGINE

◇

When I eat out, I often go for Moroccan food. It's so flavourful and usually pretty healthy. One of the most popular dishes at my local Moroccan restaurant is a tagine. It gets its name from the traditional earthen vessel in which the food is cooked. Don't worry, you won't need to go out and buy a new pot; my variation can be baked in any ovensafe dish or a slow cooker. Simply throw everything together in the morning for an amazing dinner at the end of the day.

---

serves 4

900g stewing lamb, diced

Sea salt and freshly ground black pepper

1 onion, chopped

6–8 carrots, chopped

1 x 400g tin chickpeas, rinsed and drained (optional)

2 garlic cloves, crushed

2 tablespoons ground ginger

2 tablespoons ground cumin

2 tablespoons paprika

2 tablespoons onion powder

2 tablespoons garlic powder

80g dried apricots, halved

90g pitted prunes

A handful of fresh parsley, chopped, for garnish (optional)

Herbed Quinoa Pilaf (see page 158) or Good Gut Green Rice (see page 159), to serve

TO COOK IN A SLOW COOKER:
Combine all the ingredients except the parsley in a 6-litre slow cooker and add 500–700ml of water, to generously cover. Cover and cook on high for 4–5 hours, or on low for 7.

TO COOK ON THE HOB:
Pat the lamb dry and season with salt and pepper. Heat a large saucepan over medium heat. Add the lamb and cook until browned on all sides, about 10 minutes. Transfer the meat to a plate and set aside.

Put the chopped onion and a dash of salt in the same pan and cook until translucent, 5–7 minutes. Add the carrots, chickpeas (if using), garlic, spices, apricots and prunes and cook, stirring, for a further 3 minutes.

Return the meat to the slow cooker and add 500–700ml of water to generously cover. Bring the water to the boil, then reduce the heat to maintain a simmer and cook uncovered for 1 hour.

Garnish with fresh parsley and serve with herbed quinoa or green rice.

SURF-OR-TURF FAJITAS

TGIFriday's sizzling fajitas were my favourite thing growing up. I still love this DIY-style meal – anytime I get to assemble my plate exactly the way I want it I'm happy! For this reason, homemade fajitas easily fit the Good Gut Rule of Five – you can load up on the veggies, protein and healthy fats to create the ideal plate combo. Plus, I find this type of dish forces me to s-l-o-w down, which is a key part of my approach to healthy weight loss.

serves 8–10

3 tablespoons tamari or coconut aminos

Juice of 2 limes

2 tablespoons olive oil, plus more for
 cooking

1 tablespoon ground cumin, plus
 ½ teaspoon ground cumin

2 tablespoons coconut sugar

4 garlic cloves, crushed

700g beef brisket or peeled and deveined
 prawns

1 red onion, sliced

3 red, yellow or orange peppers, cored,
 deseeded and sliced

½ teaspoon chilli powder

1 teaspoon dried oregano

1 teaspoon sea salt

¼ teaspoon cayenne pepper

1 beef tomato, diced

Guacamole (shopbought is okay)

Natural yogurt, for serving

Fresh herbs, chopped, for serving

In a large bowl, combine the tamari, lime juice, 2 tablespoons of olive oil, 1 tablespoon cumin, coconut sugar and garlic.

Add the beef or prawns to the bowl, cover and marinate in the refrigerator. If using steak, leave it to sit for 1–2 hours. If using prawns, leave them to marinate for only 10–15 minutes.

In a large frying pan, heat a little olive oil over medium heat. Add the onion and cook, stirring, for 5 minutes. Add the peppers, chilli powder, oregano, salt, cayenne and remaining cumin and cook for 3 minutes more.

Add the beef or prawns and as much of the marinade as you'd like and cook, stirring, until the meat is cooked to your liking or the prawns are pink and opaque. If using beef, remove it from the pan and let it rest for a few minutes, then slice it into thin strips across the grain.

Top with the diced tomato, some guacamole, a dollop of yogurt and some chopped herbs and serve in tortillas or over rice or greens.

◇

ROCKSTAR VEGGIE BURGERS

I've been on the hunt for a good homemade veggie burger recipe for years. I shared a black-bean burger variation in my first book, but I wanted to come up with a bean-free option, since legumes can be difficult for people to digest. These cauliflower and sweet-potato burgers are loaded with digestion-boosting herbs and spices. Plus they pack in a ton of veggies. Serve them on a burger bun of choice, atop a salad or on a Good Gut Rule of Five bowl (see pages 26–7).

---

serves 6

Coconut or avocado oil spray

1 head of cauliflower, cored and chopped

4 small sweet potatoes, peeled and chopped

1 tablespoon coconut oil, melted

½ teaspoon sea salt, plus more as needed

Freshly ground black pepper

A handful of fresh coriander, finely chopped

½ teaspoon ground cumin

Juice of ½ lime

½ teaspoon chilli powder

½ teaspoon garlic powder

2 avocados, smashed

QUICK-PICKLED ONIONS

1 medium red onion, thinly sliced

80ml red wine vinegar or apple cider vinegar

First pickled the onion. Cover the onion with the vinegar and leave it to sit for at least 15 minutes, then drain. Preheat the oven to 220ºC/gas mark 7. Line a baking tray with waxed paper or spray with coconut or avocado oil spray.

In a large bowl, toss the cauliflower, sweet potatoes in the coconut oil, then transfer to the baking tray, season with salt and pepper and roast for 25–35 minutes until golden brown. Leave to cool slightly.

Transfer the roasted cauliflower and sweet potatoes to a food-processor and pulse until mostly smooth (or mash in a bowl using a fork). Transfer to a bowl and add the coriander, cumin, lime juice, chilli powder and garlic powder. Mix to incorporate.

Form the mixture into patties about 1cm thick and place them on the baking tray you used for the veg. Bake for 30 minutes, flipping the burgers once halfway through – you may need to use two spatulas when flipping. Finish the burgers by grilling on high for 5–10 minutes.

To serve, top each burger smashed avocado some pickled onions.

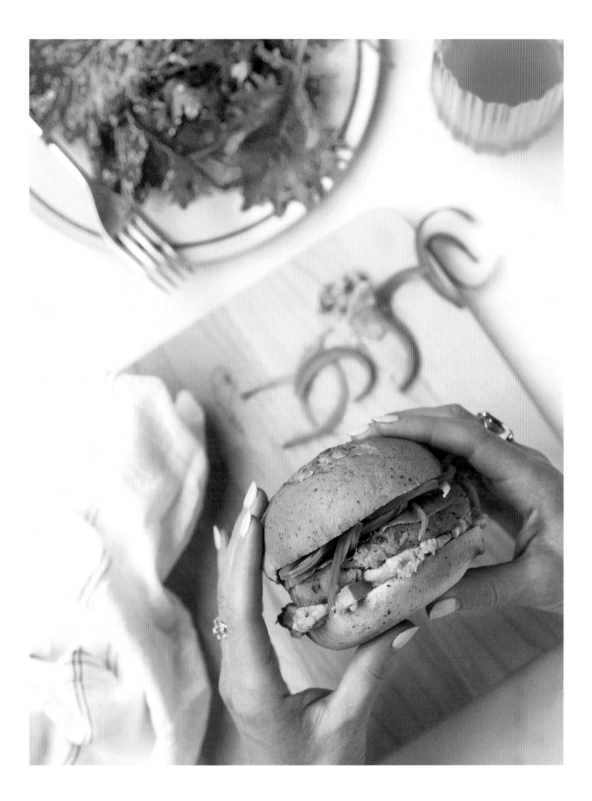

THE
SIMPLEST
SALMON

◇

My sweet mother-in-law is an amazing cook and I always turn to her for easy fish recipes that wow. Whether you're throwing together a 20-minute week-night meal or want to impress guests at a dinner party without spending hours in the kitchen, this salmon is a go-to. Salmon is a dense source of protein and healthy fat, both key for gut health and weight loss. This pairs beautifully with some simply grilled asparagus and the Good Gut Green Rice on page 159.

serves 3–4

2 tablespoons melted ghee or butter,
   cooled to room temperature
450g skin-on salmon fillet
Sea salt and freshly ground black pepper
50g flaked almonds, very lightly toasted
Drizzle of raw honey, optional

Preheat the oven to 200°C/gas mark 6. Use some of the ghee or butter to grease a large baking dish.

Put the salmon in the baking dish. Rub the rest of the ghee or butter on top of the salmon and season generously with salt and pepper. Cover it with the toasted almonds.

Bake for 12 minutes. Remove from the oven and, if using, drizzle the honey over the entire fillet. Return to the oven and cook another 3–8 minutes (depending on thickness of the fish). Check for doneness by flaking with a fork – the salmon should break, but not fall apart. The salmon will continue to cook a little on its own after you remove it from the oven, so you don't want it to dry out. Serve and eat!

VEGGIE-PACKED MEATBALLS

◇

Meatballs are the ultimate meal prep item. Whether you're using turkey, lamb, beef, pork or fish (yes, fish works well here!), these can be used in so many ways. Pair them with a salad and pre-roasted root veggies and you have a meal in 15 minutes or less. And as a bonus, this take on the classic has way more veggies (are you noticing a trend here?), without compromising the distinctive Italian flavour profile.

serves 4–6

Oil, for greasing (optional)

450g minced beef, turkey, chicken, pork or fish

About 350g grated veggies, e.g. courgette, carrot, onion, fennel

1 teaspoon sea salt

2 large eggs

2 tablespoons Italian seasoning (see note)

Preheat the oven to 180°C/gas mark 4. Line a rimmed baking tray with greaseproof paper or grease it with a little oil.

Combine all the ingredients in a bowl and mix until well incorporated.

Form the meat mixture into balls of roughly 5cm in diameter and arrange them on the baking tray.

Bake for 15–20 minutes, or until well browned.

note

IN PLACE OF THE ITALIAN SEASONING, MAKE YOUR OWN BLEND BY COMBINING CHOPPED FRESH ROSEMARY, FRESH THYME LEAVES, CRUSHED GARLIC, FRESHLY GROUND BLACK PEPPER AND CRUSHED CHILLIES. YOU'LL NEED ABOUT 3 TABLESPOONS.

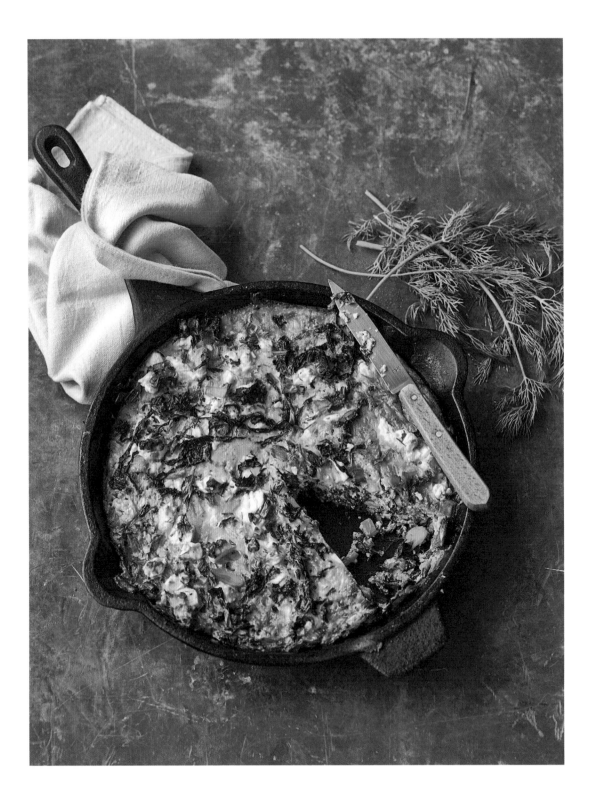

◇

KALE SPANAKOPITA

Yes, I said kale and yes, I said spanakopita. This version of the classic Greek dish is adapted from Doris Choi's amazing recipe and skips the filo pastry in favour of tons of kale and lots of fresh herbs and spices. A cast-iron frying pan works best here as it's naturally non-stick and food stays hotter than in other types of pots and pans. Plus, cooking with cast iron adds iron (a nutrient many of us are low or deficient in) to your dish.

---

serves about 6

1 teaspoon unsalted butter, olive oil or coconut oil

3 garlic cloves, crushed

½ onion, chopped

1 fennel bulb, chopped

½ teaspoon sea salt

¼ teaspoon freshly ground black pepper

5 large eggs

2 spring onions, chopped

Large handful of fresh dill, chopped

Large handful of fresh parsley, chopped

110–175g feta cheese, crumbled

Leaves from 1 bunch of kale, finely chopped

Preheat the oven to 180°C/gas mark 4.

In a large cast-iron frying pan, melt the butter, or heat the oil, over medium heat. Add the garlic, onion and fennel, season with the salt and pepper and cook, stirring, for 5–7 minutes.

In a large bowl, whisk together the eggs, spring onions, dill, parsley and feta. Set aside.

Add the chopped kale to the vegetables and onions in the frying pan and continue cooking, stirring, for 5 minutes, or until the kale has wilted.

Slowly add the vegetable mixture to the bowl with the egg mixture, stir to combine and transfer everything back to the frying pan.

Put the frying pan in the oven and bake for 15–25 minutes. The spanakopita is done when the centre has set and the edges begin to brown.

Serve immediately or leave to cool and store in an airtight container in the fridge for meals throughout the week.

tip

THIS RECIPE REHEATS BEAUTIFULLY AND MAKES A PERFECT PARTY APPETISER, BREAKFAST, LUNCH, DINNER OR SNACK – IT'S TRULY MULTIPURPOSE.

◇

AMAZING MARBELLA, TWO WAYS

Growing up, I would thumb through my mum's cookbook collection and find one of my favourites, The Silver Palate Cookbook by Julee Rosso and Sheila Lukins. As an incredible entertainer, then and now, my mum would often look here for inspiration. Chicken Marbella is one of the most famous dishes from that book, with its special combination of sweet prunes and briny capers and olives. This adaptation is great for batch cooking or for entertaining.

---

serves 6–8

1–2 chickens (about 2.25kg total),
   quartered, or about 700g firm tofu

60ml olive oil

60ml apple cider vinegar

60g pitted prunes

50g pitted Spanish green olives

40g capers in brine, drained

3 bay leaves

1 head garlic, cloves separated and
   smashed or crushed

4 tablespoons fresh oregano, chopped, or
   2 tablespoons dried

2 teaspoons sea salt

Pinch freshly ground black pepper

1–2 tablespoons coconut sugar

120ml white wine

1–2 tablespoons chopped fresh parsley

If using chicken, pat the pieces dry and place them in a large bowl. If using tofu, drain the tofu blocks and wrap them in kitchen paper. Put them in a roasting pan and place a small plate on top of each. Place a weight (e.g. a book, heavy bowl, or tin of tomatoes) on top of each plate to apply pressure. Set aside for at least 1 hour.

In a large bowl, combine the olive oil, vinegar, prunes, olives, capers, bay leaves, garlic, oregano, salt and pepper. Add the chicken or tofu to the mixture. Cover with clingfilm and leave to marinate in the fridge for 6–24 hours.

When you're ready to cook, preheat the oven to 180°C/gas mark 5.

Transfer the chicken or tofu to a roasting pan and pour the marinade over the top. Sprinkle with the coconut sugar then pour over the wine.

Bake for 1–1 1/2 hours. The chicken is done when the thigh pieces yield clear golden (not pink) juices when pricked with a fork. The tofu is done when the top begins to brown.

Garnish with the parsley and serve.

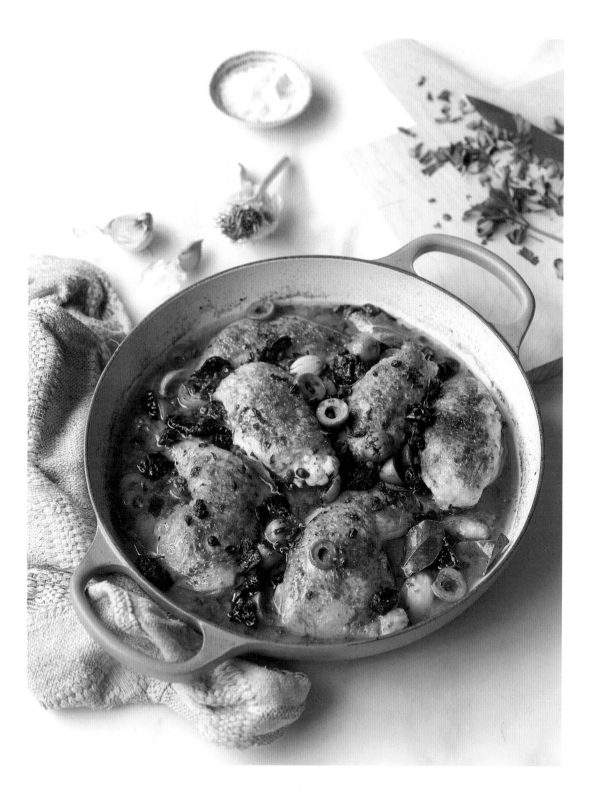

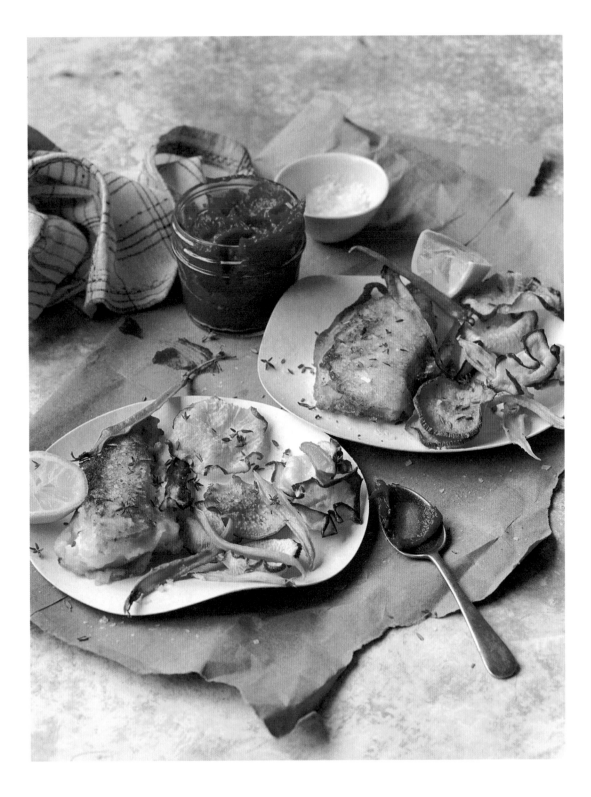

KOMBUCHA-BATTERED FISH

Fish and chips is a classic comfort meal, but not exactly weight-loss friendly dish. The solution? Use kombucha and a gluten-free flour and shallow-fry instead of deep-frying. Serve with my Root Veggie Crisps and Amped-Up Ketchup (see page 132) and a side salad for a great family meal that's healthy, too.

serves 3

450g firm white fish fillet, cut into large 'fingers' and seasoned with salt

225–275g plain kombucha

225g brown or white rice flour

1 teaspoon baking powder

Pinch of sea salt

3 tablespoons coconut oil

Vinegar of your choice or fresh lemon juice

Fresh thyme leaves, to serve

In a bowl, combine the kombucha, rice flour, baking powder and salt.

In a medium non-stick frying pan, melt the coconut oil over medium heat. Test the oil by dropping a little batter into the pan; if it sizzles, you're ready to sear.

Dip the fish 'fingers' in the batter, shake off any excess and carefully place in the hot oil. Do not crowd the pan.

Cook the fish for 2–3 minutes on each side until lightly browned. Repeat with the remaining fish.

Serve with Amped-Up Ketchup and Root Veggie Chips (see page 132).

◇

AMPED-UP KETCHUP

---

serves 6–8

1 x 200g jar organic
tomato purée

2–3 tablespoons pure
maple syrup

1 tablespoon
sauerkraut juice
(from a jar or

container of prepared
sauerkraut)

Pinch of cayenne
pepper

¾ teaspoon sea salt

1 small garlic clove,
crushed

Combine all the ingredients in a bowl and mix well.

Transfer the ketchup to a sterilised jar that leaves a little room for expansion at the top and seal. Leave to ferment at room temperature for a minimum of 24 hours and up to 3 days. You can taste the ketchup after the first 24 hours and see if it's tangy enough for your taste buds. If not, leave it to ferment a while longer, unscrewing the lid once a day to let any gas escape.

When it's fermented to your liking, transfer the jar to the fridge. The ketchup will keep for up to 3 weeks.

◇

ROOT VEGGIE CRISPS

---

serves 4–6

2 golden beetroot,
peeled and thinly
sliced

1 small swede or
jicama, peeled and
thinly sliced

1–2 tablespoons
avocado oil or
coconut oil

Sea salt and freshly
ground black pepper

Preheat the oven to 110°C/gas mark ¼.

Combine the root veggies in a large bowl and toss with the avocado oil.

Arrange the veggies on a baking tray in a single layer (use another baking tray if you need to so that the veggie chips don't overlap).

Roast in the oven for 1–1½ hours, until browned and some of the edges start to curl.

Remove from the oven and season with salt and pepper.

SPAGHETTI SQUASH BOLOGNESE

◇

When I'm craving pasta, I often find that what I really want is heaps of tomato sauce, so I'll make spaghetti squash in the style of classic Bolognese. I switch the ratio so there's about twice as much veg as meat and, suddenly, what used to be a classic 'diet no-no' food becomes a comforting weight-loss-friendly week-night dinner.

serves 8

Coconut oil

1 spaghetti squash, halved

Sea salt and freshly ground black pepper

2 tablespoons extra-virgin olive oil

1 onion, chopped

2 garlic cloves, finely chopped

Leaves from 2 sprigs of rosemary, finely
   chopped or left whole

3 celery stalks, chopped

3 medium carrots, chopped

700g minced meat (turkey, beef or lamb)

2 x 400g tins chopped tomatoes

Pinch of crushed chillies

Preheat the oven to 190°C/gas mark 5.

Rub coconut oil on the cut sides of the squash and season with salt and pepper. Set the squash cut-side down on a baking tray. Bake for 30–45 minutes, or until fork-tender. Use a fork to scrape the squash flesh into strands; discard the skin.

While the squash is cooking, heat the olive oil in a large frying pan over medium heat. Add the onion and garlic with pinch of salt and cook, stirring, until the onion is translucent, about 10 minutes.

Add the rosemary, celery and carrots, season with a bit more salt and black pepper and cook, stirring, for 5 minutes more. Add the minced meat and cook until browned, about 7–10 minutes.

Add the chopped tomatoes and season with salt, black pepper and the crushed chillies. Simmer the sauce for 5–10 minutes.

Serve the sauce over cooked spaghetti squash immediately, or reduce the heat to maintain a simmer, cover and keep warm for up to 20 minutes before serving.

SPAGHETTI SWITCH-UP

VEGETARIAN Swap the meat in the recipe on page 133 for some vegetarian-style meatballs or crumbled tempeh.

PESTO PERFECTION Mix roasted spaghetti squash with 1 or 2 spiralised courgettes. Toss with pesto and top with sautéed prawns.

PUT AN EGG ON IT While you're cooking the spaghetti squash, roast some cherry tomatoes tossed in olive oil on a separate tray. Top the squash with the tomatoes, a poached egg, some snipped chives and black pepper.

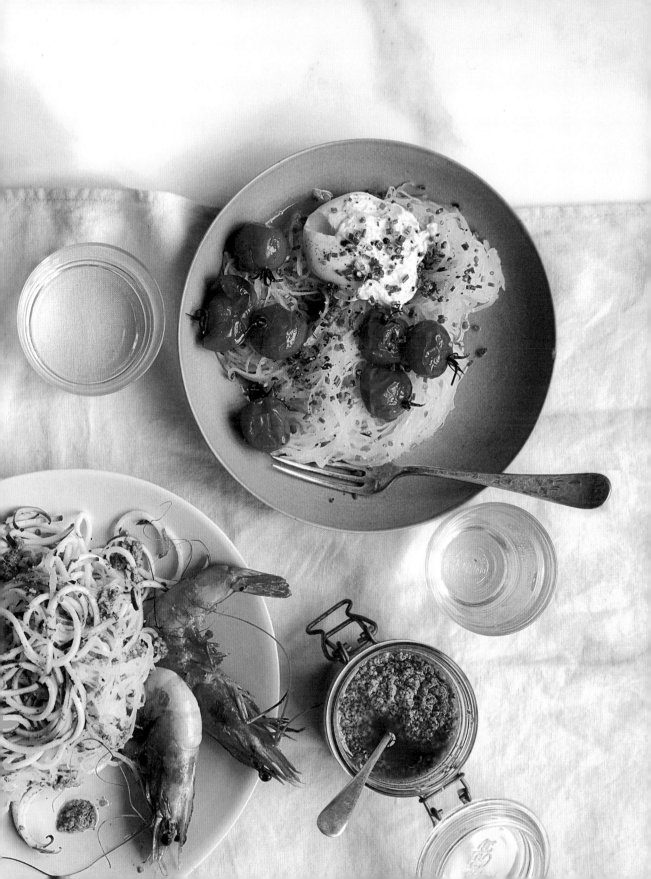

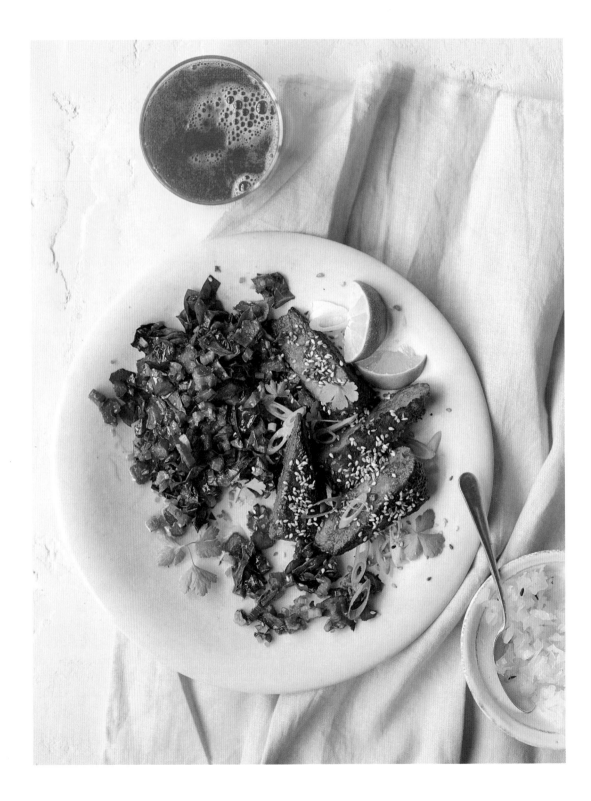

◇

SAVOURY SUNFLOWER BUTTER TEMPEH

Tempeh is a weekly staple in my diet, as it's a gut-friendly vegetarian protein. I usually simply sear it in coconut oil and tamari, but when I want to mix it up, I make this version, which tastes even better than Chinese takeout. You can add this tempeh to a salad, or serve it with stir-fry veggies and rice (or cauliflower rice) for a complete meal.

serves 2–3

¼ teaspoon crushed chillies

2 tablespoons toasted sesame oil

2 tablespoons sunflower seed butter (or almond or peanut butter)

2 tablespoons tamari or coconut aminos

Juice of 1 lime

3 tablespoons pure maple syrup

275g tempeh, cut into 2cm triangles or sliced

OPTIONAL GARNISHES

Spring onions, sliced

Sesame seeds

Chopped fresh coriander and/or parsley

Combine all the ingredients except the tempeh and garnishes in a medium bowl and mix well. Add the tempeh and turn to coat well in the marinade. Cover and marinate in the fridge for at least 2 hours and up 24 hours.

When ready to cook the tempeh, preheat the oven to 190°C/gas mark 5 and line a baking tray with greaseproof paper.

Remove the tempeh from the marinade and arrange on the prepared baking tray in an even layer. Reserve the marinade.

Bake the tempeh for 20–30 minutes, or until golden brown and caramelised. Remove the baking tray from the oven and brush the tempeh with the reserved marinade.

Garnish as wished and serve.

tip

SUNFLOWER SEED BUTTER IS A NICE ALLERGEN-FREE ALTERNATIVE TO NUT BUTTERS.

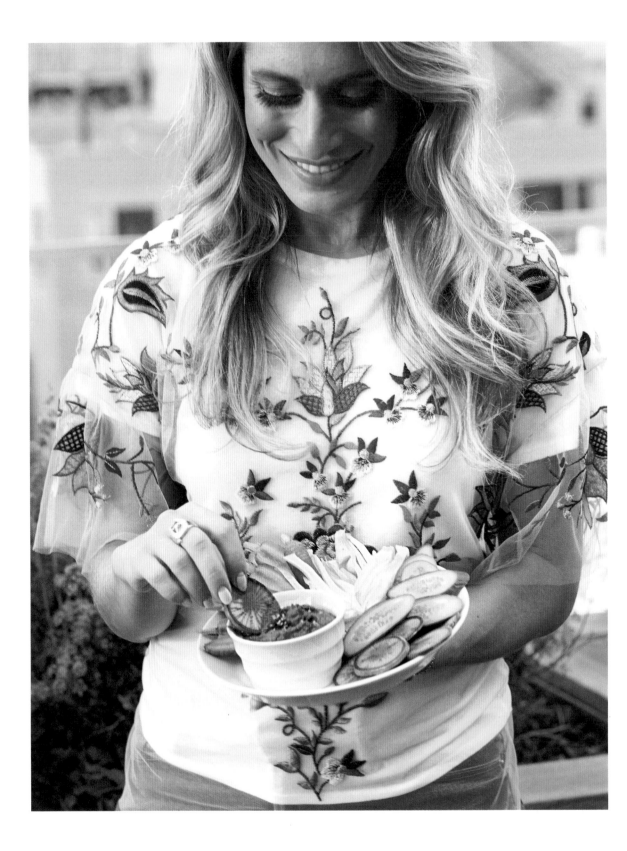

SNACKS, SIDES AND SHAREABLES

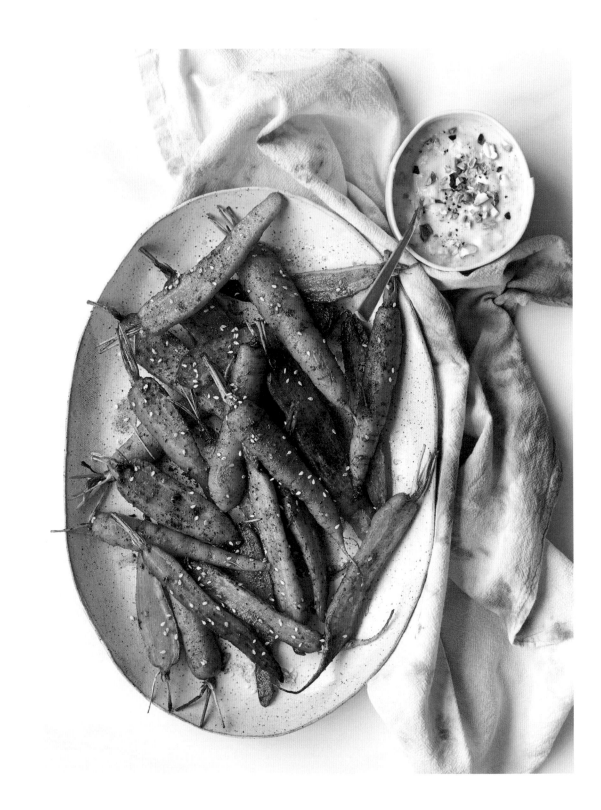

◇

ZA'ATAR-
ROASTED
CARROTS

When I tested these babies, they didn't even make it to the table – my family ate almost all of them off the tray! When you roast carrots, they become super sweet, and if you add savoury za'atar spice, nutty pistachios and aromatic cardamom cream, you have the ultimate side dish or appetiser.

---

serves 4

450g carrots, cut into sticks
   or halved lengthways
1–2 tablespoons coconut oil, melted
½ teaspoon sea salt
½ teaspoon ground cumin
2 tablespoons za'atar (see note)
About 150g natural goats'-milk yogurt
1 teaspoon ground cardamom
30g pistachios, chopped

Preheat the oven to 220°C/gas mark 7.

In a large bowl, toss the carrots with the coconut oil and place on a rimmed baking try. Sprinkle with the salt, cumin and za'atar.

Roast in the oven for 25–35 minutes, or until browned to your liking.

Meanwhile, in a small bowl, stir together the yogurt and cardamom.

Garnish the carrots with the cardamom cream and chopped pistachios.

tip

THE SPICED ROASTED CARROTS ARE WONDERFUL EVEN WITHOUT THE PISTACHIOS AND CARDAMOM CREAM, IF YOU ARE SHORT ON TIME OR INGREDIENTS!

note

ZA'ATAR IS A SPICE BLEND MADE WITH THYME, DRIED SUMAC, SESAME SEEDS AND OFTEN OTHER HERBS AND SPICES, TOO. YOU CAN FIND IT AT MIDDLE EASTERN GROCERS OR ONLINE, OR MAKE YOUR OWN BLEND AT HOME.

◇

RUBY RED SAUERKRAUT

While both red and green cabbage are good for you, red cabbage actually contains twice as much vitamin C and more inflammation-fighting phytonurients. Red cabbage also has a slightly different flavour which makes this ruby sauerkraut a bit more zippy than a more traditional recipe.

---

makes about 1 litre

1 large head of red cabbage, two outer leaves removed and reserved, remainder finely shredded

1 tablespoon sea salt or Himalayan pink salt, plus more if needed

1 medium beetroot, sliced into thin strips

Filtered water

In a large bowl, mix the shredded cabbage and salt by hand, until the cabbage starts to get all juicy and you have liquid pooling at the bottom of the bowl. You'll need to spend a bit of time on this. Taste it throughout; it should taste very, very salty. Add the beetrootroot and mix again.

Pack the veggies into a sterilised 1½-litre preserving jar. You'll need to stuff the jar with a few centimetres of the veggies then pack it tightly down before adding more and repeating. Liquid should cover the veggies at each stage of the packing and layering. Pack the veggies to within a couple of centimetres

of the top of the jar, making sure they remain covered with the liquid. Add a splash of filtered water if needed to keep them covered (or you may need a smaller jar, depending on the quantity of cabbage used).

Fold one of the reserved outer cabbage leaves and place it over the veggies in the jar to further press the veggies below the liquid. Seal the jar loosely and leave at room temperature in a cool, dark place to ferment for a week or more. 'Burp' the sauerkraut every day or two. (To do this, simply unscrew the lid and allow the air to escape, then seal again.) You may need to pack the veggies down with your fist again if they're not covered with liquid.

After about a week, taste the sauerkraut. It should taste sour and slightly salty with a tangy flavour and have a nice but strong aroma. If it tastes good, it's good. If it tastes bad, you may need to scrape off the top layer and see if the sauerkraut tastes better beneath the liquid. Ferment it for as long as you like! I find that anything between 10 days and 1 month tastes great, but you can let some ferments go a year or more. Once the taste is to your liking, seal the jar tightly and store in the fridge.

◇

PLANTAIN CRISPS

Plantains are an underused source of prebiotic fibre (that's the fibre that feeds those good probiotic bugs in your gut). Serve these with hummus (try my Beetroot Hummus, see page 148), black bean dip, or eat them straight up.

serves 4

2 plantains (green will
  be starchier; yellow
  will be sweeter), thinly
  sliced on a mandoline
  into strips or rounds

2 teaspoons coconut oil
  or coconut oil spray
1 teaspoon sea salt
Squeeze of fresh lime
  juice

Preheat the oven to 190°C/gas mark 5. Line a baking tray with greaseproof paper.

Brush the sliced plantains with coconut oil or spray with coconut oil spray. Arrange them on the prepared baking tray and sprinkle with the salt. Roast for 15–20 minutes.

Squeeze lime juice over the top before serving.

◇

SUPERFOOD SEAWEED CRISPS

If there was ever a yummy superfood snack, this is it. Seaweed is high in natural minerals, including folate, calcium, magnesium, zinc, iron, selenium and iodine, which is crucial for proper thyroid function and metabolism.

serves 1–2

1 teaspoon coconut oil
1 package whole leaf
  dulse

Sea salt

In a frying pan, melt the coconut oil over medium heat.

Add the dulse and cook until crisp, about 5 minutes.

Finish with a sprinkle of sea salt and eat!

tip

DULSE IS A BURGUNDY-COLOURED SEAWEED
THAT'S USUALLY SOLD DRIED.

PRETTY-IN-PINK FERMENTED RADISHES

Brined cut or whole veggies are some of the easiest fermented foods to make and they taste seriously gourmet. These fermented radishes are awesome in salads, or as part of a Go with Your Gut Rule of Five plate. If you've been on the fence about fermenting your own veggies, start here.

makes about 350g

3 bunches of radishes, thinly sliced

1 teaspoon pink peppercorns

A large handful of fresh dill, chopped

1 teaspoon sea salt

Filtered water

1 kale or cabbage leaf

Combine the radishes, peppercorns, dill and salt in a large bowl. Squish by hand until the radishes have released their liquid.

Transfer the radish mixture to a sterilised 350ml preserving jar and press down so that the liquid covers the radishes, adding some filtered water to top up the level if necessary.

Place the kale or cabbage leaf over the radishes so they stay submerged.

Seal the jar loosely and set aside in a cool, dark place to ferment. 'Burp' the radishes once a day for the first 3 days. (Simply unscrew the lid and allow the air to escape, then seal again.)

note

MAKE SURE YOU USE A FRESH, CLEAN FORK EVERY TIME YOU SCOOP RADISHES FROM THE JAR. THIS KEEPS THE UNIQUE BACTERIA IN YOUR MOUTH FROM MIXING AND MULTIPLYING IN YOUR JAR.

Ferment the radishes for 1–3 weeks. Begin tasting after a week. When they are fermented to your liking, move them to the fridge. They will keep in the fridge for up to 6 months.

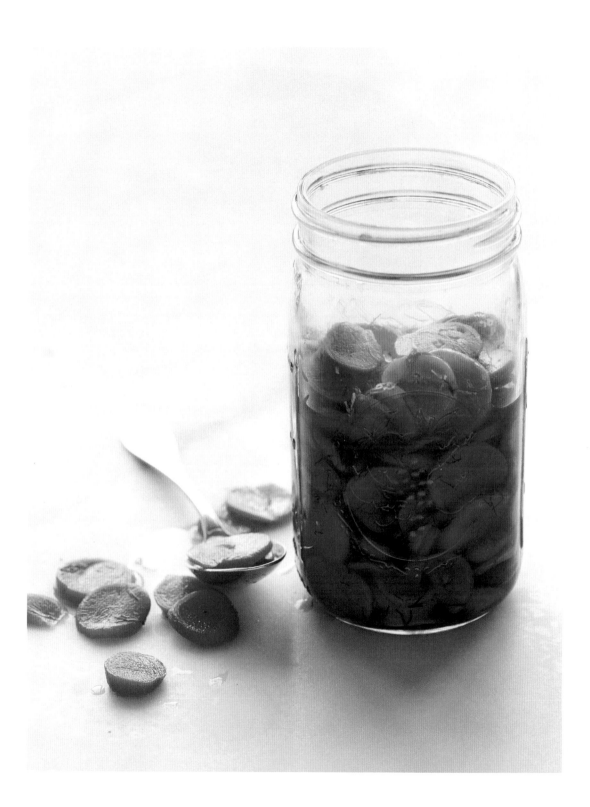

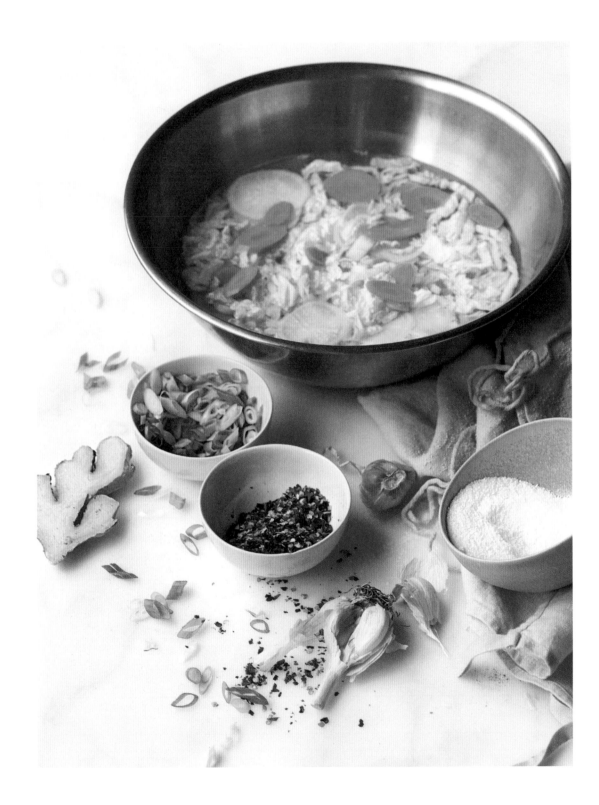

◇

EASY
KIMCHI

Add a couple of spoonfuls of this spicy and exotic ferment to your next stir-fry or Bibimbap Breakfast Bowl (see page 78), or mix some into a lunchtime salad for a serious kick of flavour. The best part about making your own kimchi is that you can adjust the level of spiciness to your liking by using more – or, in my case, less – chilli flakes.

---

makes two 2-litre jars

1 head of Chinese leaf, outer leaves removed and
*   reserved, remainder shredded*
2 carrots, cut into ribbons or thinly sliced on an
*   angle*
1 daikon radish (about 15cm long), thinly sliced
Filtered water
1 tablespoon sea salt
1 bunch of spring onions, sliced
4 garlic cloves, thinly sliced
2–3cm piece of ginger, peeled and grated
1–3 teaspoons crushed chillies

Place the Chinese leaf, carrot and daikon in a large bowl. Add filtered water to cover, stir in the salt and cover with clingfilm. Leave to sit at room temperature for 24–48 hours.

Pour off most of the water; the vegetables need to be wet but not drowning in liquid. Add the spring onions, garlic, ginger and 1 teaspoon of the crushed chillies and mix together. Taste and add more crushed chillies if you want more kick.

Transfer the vegetable mixture into two sterilised 2-litre jars and push down to immerse the veggies in the liquid. Add filtered water, if needed, to cover the veggies and top with one of the reserved leaves.

Seal the jar loosely and set aside in a cool, dark place to ferment. 'Burp' the kimchi daily for the first week and once every few days thereafter.

Ferment for 1–4 weeks. Taste the kimchi every few days as it ferments. When the flavour is to your liking, seal the jar and store in the fridge for up to 6 months.

note

TO BURP YOUR KIMCHI, SIMPLY UNSCREW THE LID AND ALLOW THE AIR TO ESCAPE, THEN SEAL AGAIN.

◇

BEAUTIFUL BEETROOT HUMMUS

This beetroot version of classic hummus is bright and beautiful, and a fun way to get kids (and indeed anyone) to eat more veggies. Who wouldn't want to eat cucumber rounds or celery sticks dipped in something hot pink? It's equally delicious spread on toast, or added to salads and bowl meals instead of a dressing.

---

makes about 500g

1 small beetroot (or purchase pre-cooked
   beetroot for a shortcut)
1 x 400g tin chickpeas, drained and rinsed
2 garlic cloves, crushed
2 tablespoons tahini
60ml extra-virgin olive oil, plus more for
   drizzling
Juice of 1 lemon
1 tablespoon ground cumin
1 teaspoon sea salt
Pinch of freshly ground black pepper
Pinch of cayenne pepper
Fresh parsley, for garnish
Crudités, bread and/or crackers, to serve

Preheat the oven to 200°C/gas mark 6.

Wrap the beetroot in foil and place it in a small roasting pan. Roast until fork-tender, about 25 minutes. Leave to cool.

Unwrap and chop the beetroot and place in a food-processor with the chickpeas, garlic, tahini, olive oil, lemon juice, cumin, salt and black and cayenne peppers and process until smooth. Taste and add more salt, pepper or other seasoning if needed.

Spread on a platter or spoon into a bowl, drizzle with olive oil and garnish with parsley.

Enjoy with crudités or on your favourite crackers or bread!

LOVE YOUR LIVER PÂTÉ

◇

In general, organ meats are between ten and one hundred times higher in nutrients than corresponding muscle meats; liver, in particular, is rich in vitamins A, D, E, K, B12 and folic acid, as well as copper and iron. However, liver, like so many other foods, has been slowly phased out of our everyday diets, mostly because these foods aren't 'fashionable'. Give liver a try with this rich pâté recipe.

makes about 500g

3 tablespoons ghee

1 garlic clove, crushed

1 onion, finely chopped

1 bay leaf

1 sprig of thyme

1 sprig of rosemary

1 sprig of sage

¼ teaspoon sea salt, plus more as needed

700g chicken livers, cleaned

3 tablespoons apple cider vinegar

In a large frying pan, melt the ghee over medium heat. Add the garlic, onion and herbs and season with salt. Add the livers and cook for 7–10 minutes.

Add the vinegar and cook for a further 3–5 minutes.

Remove the herbs and transfer the mixture to a blender or food-processor. Blend until smooth. If you want to thin the pâté, add up to 120ml water.

Serve immediately, or transfer to an airtight container and refrigerate for up to 1 week.

This also freezes really well. Scoop the pâté in tablespoon-sized portions onto a greaseproof-paper-lined baking tray, freeze until solid, then transfer to a zip-top bag and return to the freezer for up to 6 months.

tip

NOT USED TO EATING LIVER PÂTÉ? TRY AND THINK OF IT AS YOU WOULD HUMMUS – AS A DELICIOUS DIP OR NUTRIENT-RICH SPREAD ON YOUR SPRING GREEN SALAD WRAPS (SEE PAGE 100) OR ON YOUR SANDWICH CREATIONS.

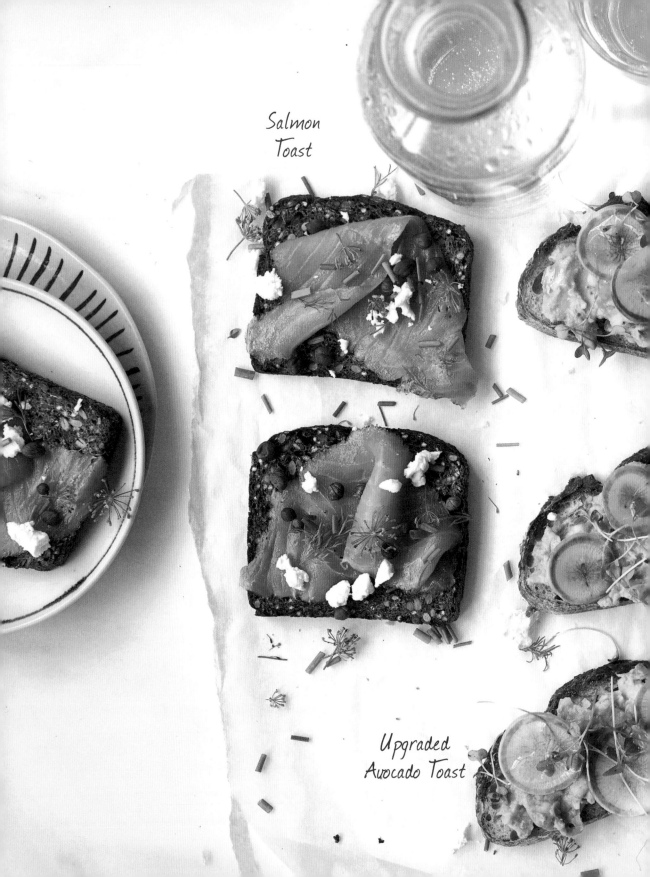

Salmon
Toast

Upgraded
Avocado Toast

SHOW ME YOUR TOASTS

TURN THE PAGE FOR MY FAVOURITE
UPGRADED TOAST IDEAS.

*Ricotta
Fig Toast*

◇

SHOW ME YOUR TOASTS

Do you remember life before avocado toast? What were we all eating (and photographing)? There's a good reason toasts are so popular: toast is really versatile and lends itself to easy meals that are also visually appealing. Here are nine upgraded toast ideas, and I'd love you to show me your best slices. Snap a photo, post to social media and tag me @RobynYoukilis so I can see your creations!

Salmon Toast – Top your toast with smoked salmon, capers, baby rocket and crumbled goats' cheese.

Upgraded Avocado Toast – Mash avocado and sauerkraut together, top with matchsticked radishes, salt and pepper and a drizzle of extra-virgin olive oil.

Ricotta Fig Toast – Spread ricotta on your toast and top with sliced figs and a drizzle of raw honey.

Sweet Potato Toast – Swap the bread for a slice of roasted sweet potato and top with almond butter, sliced pear and a sprinkle of cinnamon.

Bone Marrow Toast – Spoon bone marrow on your toast and top with quick pickled onions and fresh herbs such as thyme or parsley.

Beetroot Hummus Toast – Spread your toast with Beautiful Beetroot Hummus (see page 148) and top with spicy microgreens.

Broccoli Toast – Chop up some Crispy Coconut Broccoli (see page 156) and pile it on your toast. Garnish with lemon zest.

Liver Toast – Spread your toast with my Love Your Liver Pâté (see page 149) and top with caramelised onions and snipped fresh chives.

Mushroom Toast – Top your toast with sauteed mushrooms and chopped fresh parsley.

◇

HONEYMOON
GREENS

While I love a giant plate of straight-up steamed greens drizzled with pumpkin seed oil and sea salt, sometimes my taste buds want something a little more complex. This variation of sautéed greens does the trick – the combination of ginger, lime and shallots was inspired by my honeymoon in Bali, where these flavours were everywhere.

---

serves 2

2–3 tablespoons coconut or extra-virgin olive oil

1 bunch of dark leafy greens, stemmed, leaves chopped and dried

2 or 3 shallots, minced or grated

4cm piece of ginger, peeled and grated

Sea salt and freshly ground black pepper

Squeeze of fresh lime juice, to serve

Crushed chillies, to serve (optional)

In a large sauté pan, melt 1–2 tablespoons of the oil over medium–low heat.

Add the greens, shallots and ginger, season generously with salt and pepper and mix well.

Cook, stirring, for 5–8 minutes, until the greens are soft and have darkened in colour.

Drizzle the remaining 1 tablespoon olive or coconut oil over the greens and stir through. Scoop the greens from the pan onto two plates and serve with a squeeze of lime and a sprinkle of crushed chillies, if wished.

SOCCA FLATBREAD

◇

I love getting my creative juices flowing in the kitchen, but even after all my years in the kitchen, I'm still not much of a baker. For this reason I turn to quick breads and no-fuss flatbread recipes such as this socca. If you've discovered that gluten isn't your best friend – or are just looking for an easy starch to complete a meal – then this flatbread is for you.

---

makes 1 thick or 2 thin 25 cm flatbreads

120g chickpea flour (also labelled gram flour or besan)

1 teaspoon sea salt

2 teaspoons olive oil, plus more for drizzling

VARIATIONS

Garlic Leek: 60g chopped leek, sautéed in oil or butter; 1 tablespoon garlic powder

'Cheesy' Rosemary: 1 tablespoon nutritional yeast, 1 tablespoon chopped fresh rosemary

Cinnamon Raisin: 35g raisins, 1 teaspoon ground cinnamon

tip

POUR A THIN LAYER OF THE BATTER INTO EACH WELL OF A SILICONE MUFFIN PAN AND BAKE AS DIRECTED TO MAKE SOCCA 'CRACKERS'.

Preheat the oven to 220°C/gas mark 7.

Combine the chickpea flour, sea salt, olive oil and 240ml water in a bowl, stir and leave to sit for 30 minutes.

Place a large cast-iron frying pan in the oven to warm up for 10 minutes.

Add an additional drizzle of olive oil to the batter and then stir in the ingredients for the variation of your choice.

Add a drizzle of olive oil to the pan before adding the socca mixture. If making two thin flatbreads, carefully pour half the batter into the hot cast-iron pan in the oven. If making one thick flatbread, pour all the batter into the pan.

Bake for 10–15 minutes, or until edges begin to brown. Repeat to make a second thin pancake, if needed.

Use a spatula to remove the flatbread from the pan. Slice, serve and enjoy as is, or use it like gluten-free pizza crust.

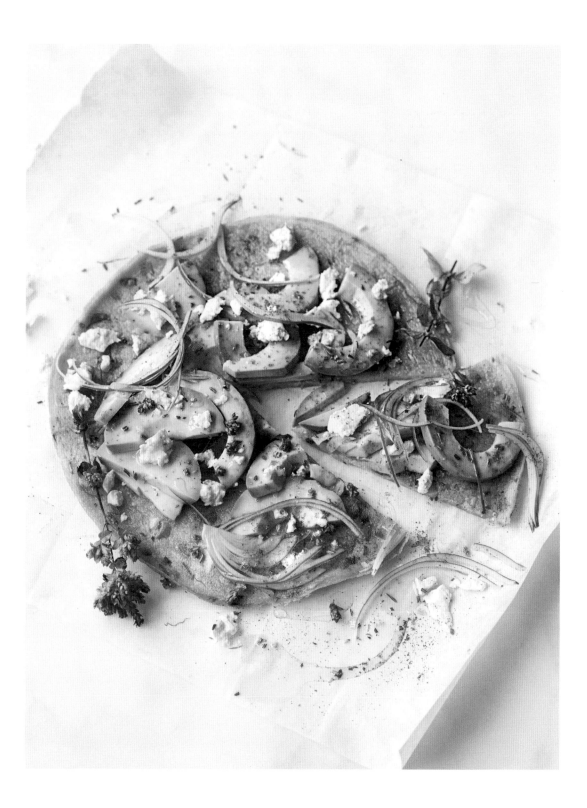

CRISPY COCONUT BROCCOLI

Toasty, crispy broccoli was a classic go-to my mum made for our family and guests, even the people who said they didn't like broccoli always loved this version. I made a few swaps to the original recipe, like adding in shredded coconut for a dose of healthy fats and fibre. It makes a great side dish for any weeknight dinner or company meal.

serves 3–4

3 heads of broccoli, chopped into florets
1 tablespoon coconut oil, melted
Sea salt and freshly ground black pepper
3 tablespoons unsweetened coconut flakes

Preheat the oven to 220ºC/gas mark 7.

Toss the broccoli with coconut oil, spread on a baking tray in a single layer and season with salt and pepper.

Bake for 25 minutes. Remove the baking tray from the oven and sprinkle the coconut flakes over the broccoli.

Bake for a further 5 minutes, until the coconut is lightly toasted, then serve hot.

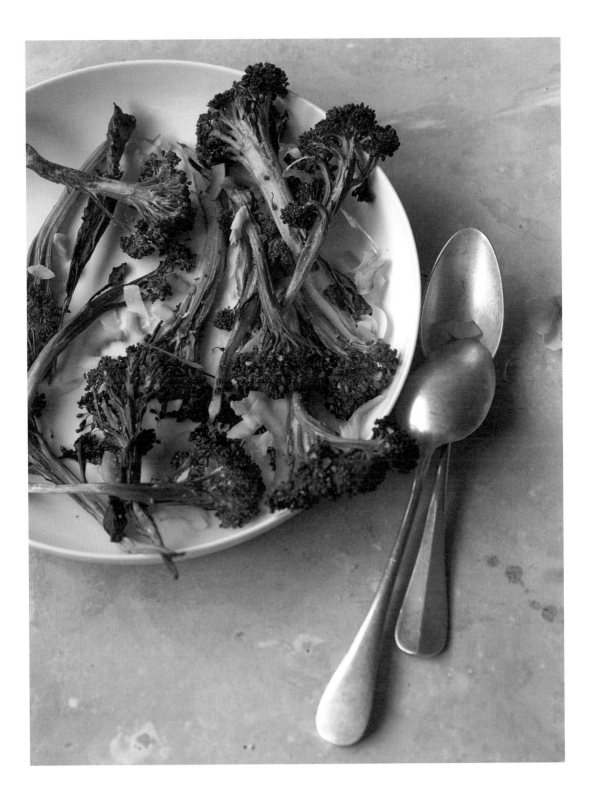

◇

HERBED
QUINOA
PILAF

I love how quinoa has its own nutty flavour, but is also enough of a blank slate to add any veggies, herbs, sauces and proteins to. Most of my recipes call for lots of herbs, and this quinoa is one easy way to use up leftovers. Make a big batch at the beginning of the week and enjoy it with your lunch or dinner.

serves 6

825ml stock or water or a mix of the two

340g quinoa

2 teaspoons sea salt

Leaves from 1 sprig of rosemary, coarsely
   chopped

2 sage leaves, finely chopped

Leaves from 3–5 sprigs of thyme

1 tablespoon ghee or coconut
   or olive oil

In a medium saucepan, bring the stock or water to the boil. Add the quinoa, salt, herbs and ghee or oil and stir. Reduce the heat to low, cover and simmer until the quinoa is cooked through and fluffy, about 20 minutes.

Remove from the heat, fluff with a fork and serve.

◇

GOOD GUT GREEN RICE

This green rice is an easy go-to grain and it pairs well with almost all my protein and veggie recipes. You can add a sauce if you want to get fancy, but it's also delicious as is.

serves 6

420g white rice (basmati or jasmine work well)

1 tablespoon ghee or coconut oil

1 leek, thinly sliced and washed well

1–2 teaspoons sea salt

Freshly ground black pepper

½ bunch of parsley, chopped

½ bunch of coriander, chopped

Rinse the rice in a fine-mesh strainer.

In a pot, melt the ghee over medium heat. Add the leek, season with the salt and pepper and cook, stirring, until soft, 5–7 minutes.

Add the rice and cook for about 1 minute.

Add 700ml water, raise the heat to medium–high and bring to the boil.

Reduce the heat to low, cover and cook until the rice is tender but not mushy, about 20 minutes.

Fluff with a fork, stir in the parsley and coriander and cover for 5 minutes more before serving.

◇

BRUSSELS SPROUTS WITH AIOLI

You heard it from me first: Brussels sprouts crisps are the new kale crisps. When I tested this recipe, I had some leftover aioli in the fridge and so the most amazing flavour combination was discovered. Try this recipe for a fancy (but easy) twist on basic roasted veggies.

serves 6

700g Brussels sprouts, trimmed and halved

3 tablespoons avocado or olive oil

1 teaspoon sea salt

Freshly ground black pepper, to taste

AIOLI

110g mayonnaise (I use ones made from
   avocado and olive oils)

1 garlic clove, crushed

½ teaspoon lemon zest

2 teaspoons fresh lemon juice

Pinch of sea salt

1 teaspoon fresh thyme leaves

Pinch of crushed chillies (optional)

Preheat the oven to 200°C/gas mark 6.

Toss the Brussels sprouts with the olive oil, salt and pepper and place on a baking tray. Bake for 35–45 minutes or until browned and crispy.

Meanwhile, mix all the aioli ingredients together in a small bowl and set aside until the Brussels sprouts are ready to enjoy.

note

THIS RECIPE CALLS FOR MAYONNAISE – CHOOSE A VERSION MADE WITHOUT SOYBEAN OR CANOLA OIL, OR CHALLENGE YOURSELF TO MAKE YOUR OWN. THE AIOLI IS ALSO DELICIOUS WITH MY KOMBUCHA-BATTERED FISH (SEE PAGE 131).

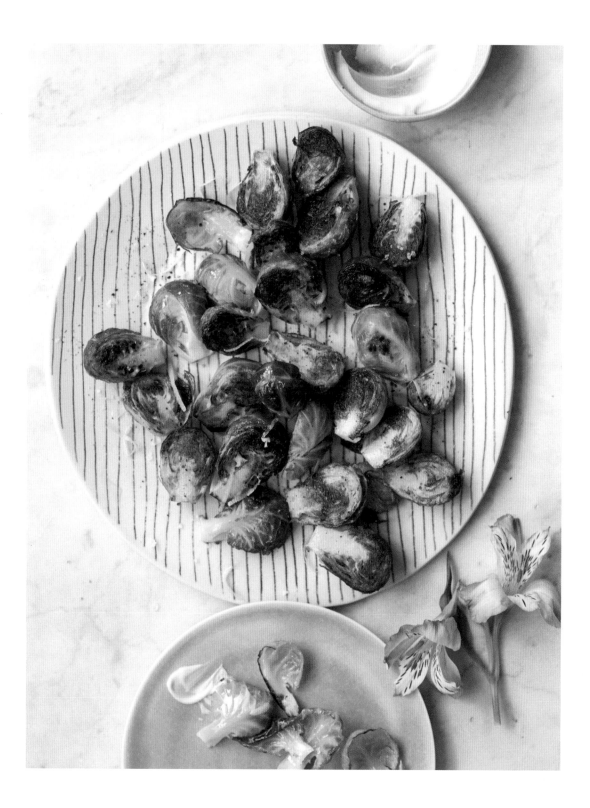

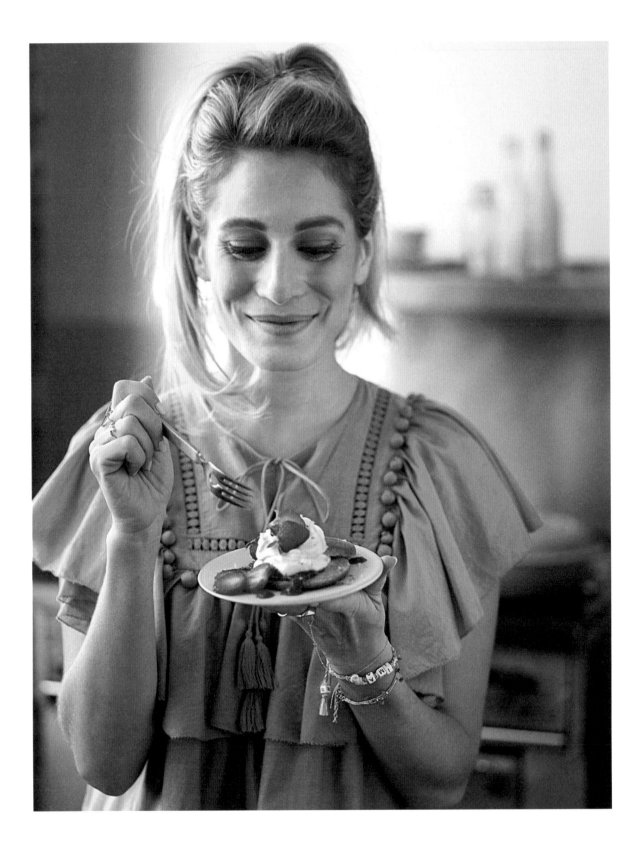

◇

SWEET
TREATS

FABULOUS FRUIT SALAD

◇

The key to this unusual fruit salad is the combination of fresh and dried fruit. It's perfect for parties and bring-and-share suppers because – let's be honest – everyone loves the person who brings a beautiful fruit salad. Bonus: the leftovers (if there are any!) are delicious in my Power Parfait (see page 36).

serves 4

2 seedless oranges, peeled, sectioned and
    cut into halves
Seeds from 1 pomegranate, or about 160g
    ready-to-serve pomegranate seeds
2 pears, cored and thinly sliced lengthways
1 apple, cored and thinly sliced
110g mix of dried apricots and Turkish figs,
    chopped
2 teaspoons raw honey
Juice of 1 lemon
A handful of fresh mint leaves, chopped

Combine the fresh and dried fruits in a bowl.

Drizzle with the honey and lemon juice, add the mint and mix together.

Leave to macerate for at least 20 minutes before serving.

GOOD-GUT JELLIES

After having my daughter, I couldn't seem to GO in the morning. What finall worked were these by-accident apple juice jellies that came together when I left my apple juice and psyllium husk mixture sitting on the counter and it thickened up. My herbalist recommended this combo and it's the only thing that go me going. On days I ate these, I went, and on days I didn't – I didn't. If you're struggling to get regular, try these as soon as possible!

serves 2

120ml organic apple juice or cider (use the most natural version you can with no added sugar)
2 tablespoons whole psyllium husk
Sprinkle of ground cinnamon (optional)

In a small jar or container, mix together the apple juice, psyllium and cinnamon, if using.

Refrigerate to firm up for 15 minutes, or leave to stand overnight. Enjoy!

tip

PSYLLIUM HUSK IS PURE SOLUBLE FIBRE AND PROMOTES EASY ELIMINATION BY PULLING WASTE OUT OF THE COLON MORE QUICKLY AND EFFICIENTLY. IT'S ALSO A PREBIOTIC FOOD, WHICH MAKES IT A GUT FRIENDLY FAVOURITE!

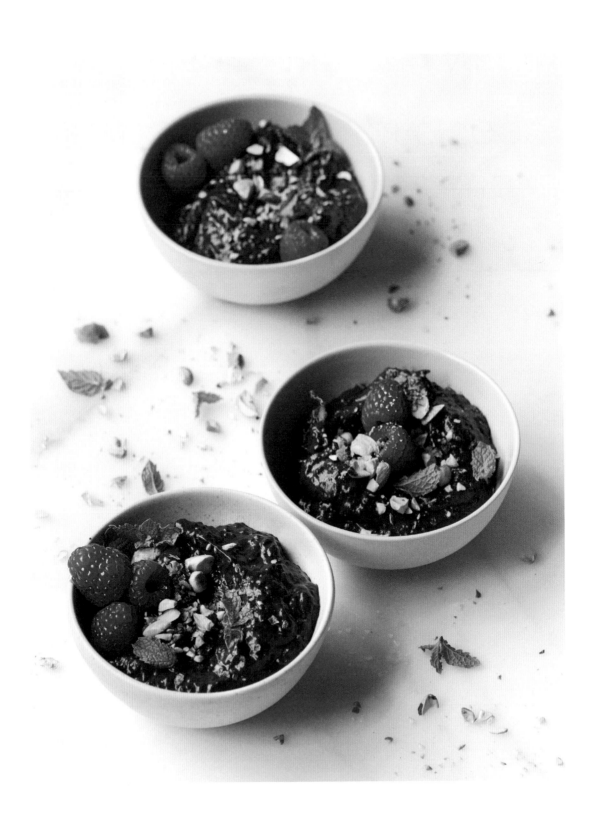

SALTED DARK CHOCOLATE PUDDING

◇

Sometimes we just need a little chocolate, and this pudding is a great treat when a square of dark chocolate won't do the job. You can't taste the avocado in here, but it makes this pudding rich and creamy. The fibre from the avocado, chia seeds and cacao will help stabilise your blood sugar, so you'll avoid the crash that's common after eating many sugar-laden desserts. And kids love it, too!

serves 2

1 ripe avocado, pitted and peeled

160ml milk of choice

2 tablespoons chia seeds

25g raw cacao powder or unsweetened
  cocoa powder

2 tablespoons date syrup (or maple syrup)

¼ teaspoon sea salt, plus more to garnish

1 teaspoon pure vanilla extract

A few fresh raspberries, crushed pistachio
  nuts, mint leaves, to decorate (optional)

Combine all the ingredients except the cayenne pepper in a blender or food-processor and blend until smooth.

Finish with a sprinkle of sea salt and garnished with a few fresh raspberries, some crushed pistachio nuts and fresh mint leaves.

◇

CHAI AND GINGER COOKIES

I love ginger cookies, but in addition to containing digestion-friendly ginger, most traditional recipes include tons of white sugar and white flour. So to avoid having to pass on them altogether, I made some swaps and came up with this version, which are as healthy as a breakfast cookie. (For a real cookie you can eat for breakfast, see page 76.). These cookies also contain turmeric, which is anti-inflammatory and great for your entire body.

makes about 16 cookies

6 tablespoons coconut oil, plus extra for
 greasing

1 teaspoon pure vanilla extract

85g molasses

200g oat flour

40g coconut sugar

2 teaspoons baking powder

1 teaspoon bicarbonate of soda

2 teaspoons grated fresh ginger

1 teaspoon grated fresh turmeric

1 teaspoon ground cinnamon

½ teaspoon ground cardamom

Pinch of sea salt

Freshly ground black pepper

60ml coconut milk or other non-dairy milk
 of choice

60g chopped crystallised ginger (optional)

Preheat the oven to 180°C/gas mark 4. Line a baking tray with greaseproof paper or grease with a little coconut oil.

In a saucepan, melt the coconut oil over medium heat. Add the vanilla and molasses and stir to combine.

In a large bowl, stir together the flour, sugar, baking powder, bicarbonate of soda, ginger, turmeric, cinnamon, cardamom, salt, and pepper to taste.

Add the melted coconut oil mixture to the bowl and mix to incorporate. Add the coconut milk and mix together. If using crystallised ginger, gently fold it into the dough. The dough will be sticky; place it in the freezer for 15 minutes so that it will be easier to work with.

Use your hands to form dough into 5cm balls. Place the balls on the baking tray about 4cm apart and flatten lightly with your palm. Bake for 8–12 minutes, or until the edges are browned and crispy.

Store the cookies in an airtight container at room temperature for up to 1 week. These also freeze well.

◇

MUM'S
HONEY
MUFFINS

This recipe was a happy accident: I was working on veggie-packed muffin for this book and ended up with a variation that tasted almost like my mum's Passover honey cake, which is out-of-this-world delicious. I still can't believe how good this recipe tastes, considering that it's almost all veggies and sweetened with just a teeny amount of raw honey.

makes about 8 muffins

Coconut oil spray

170g courgette, grated

75g carrots, grated

2 large eggs

2 tablespoons coconut oil, melted

½ teaspoon pure vanilla extract

85g raw honey

85g ground almonds

1 teaspoon ground cinnamon

½ teaspoon bicarbonate of soda

½ teaspoon baking powder

Pinch of sea salt

Preheat the oven to 180°C/gas mark 4. Grease eight wells of a standard bun tin with coconut oil spray.

Combine the shredded zucchini and carrots in a large bowl. Add the eggs, coconut oil, vanilla and honey and mix well.

In a separate medium bowl, mix together the ground almonds, cinnamon, bicarbonate of soda, baking powder and salt.

Slowly add the flour mixture to the veggie mixture and mix until combined.

Divide the batter evenly among the prepared wells of the bun tin and bake for 20–25 minutes, or until golden brown.

Cool, then store in the fridge, loosely covered, for up to 5 days.

◇

STRAWBERRY
SHORTCAKES

Strawberry shortcake is my favourite dessert in the world, so I made a healthy version I can eat more often than the real deal. This is actually three awesome recipes in one: you can use the cakes as breakfast biscuits, the frosting on healthy cupcakes and the strawberry chia jam on toast or stirred in to yogurt!

---

makes about 12 mini cakes

180g coconut oil, melted

6 large eggs

1½ teaspoons pure vanilla extract

100g coconut sugar or pure maple syrup

90g coconut flour

½ teaspoon sea salt

½ teaspoon bicarbonate of soda

JAM

150g strawberries, hulled and chopped

1 tablespoon fresh lemon juice

1 tablespoon raw honey

2 tablespoons chia seeds

FROSTING

2 x 400ml tins coconut milk, refrigerated
  overnight

85g raw honey

1 teaspoon pure vanilla extract

Pinch of sea salt

GARNISH

75g fresh strawberries, sliced

Fresh mint leaves

Preheat the oven to 180°C/gas mark 4. Grease a bun tin with a little of the coconut oil (or coconut oil spray). In a large bowl, combine the eggs, vanilla, the remaining coconut oil and the coconut sugar. Slowly add the flour, salt and bicarbonate of soda. Whisk to combine. Pour into the tin and bake for 25–30 minutes, until golden and firm on the top.

To make the jam, in a saucepan, combine the strawberries and 60ml water and cook over medium heat until the strawberries are falling apart. Add the lemon juice and honey and cook, stirring occasionally, for 5 minutes more. Remove from the heat and stir in the chia seeds. Leave to cool for at least 10 minutes.

To make the frosting, open the tins of coconut milk and pour off the clear liquid. Put the thick coconut cream in a medium bowl, add the honey, vanilla and salt and whisk until smooth.

To assemble and decorate the shortcakes, leave them to cool completely in the tins, then turn them out onto a plate or platter and slice in half.

Spread the chia jam over the bottom half of each bun. Add a large dollop of frosting and stack the other half of the bun on top. Repeat with remaining buns. Decorate with additional frosting, sliced strawberries and mint leaves. Serve and eat immediately.

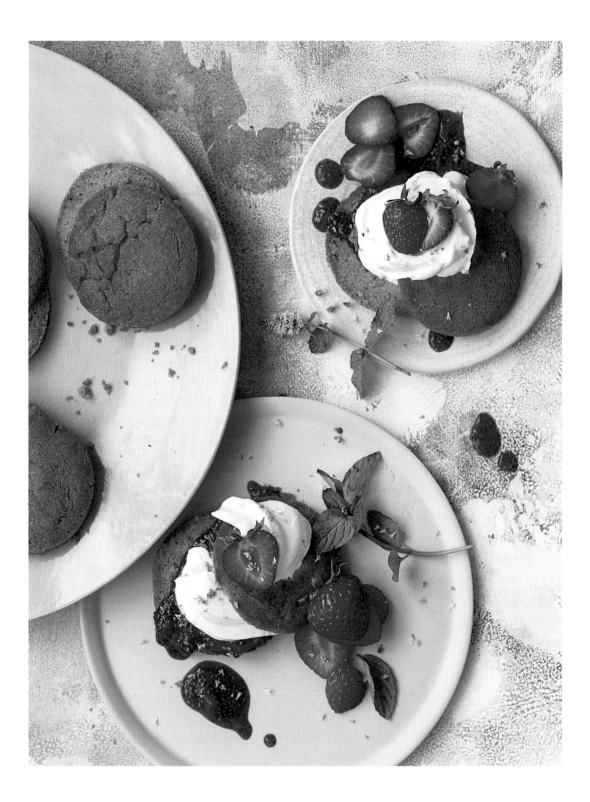

GOOD-GUT DELIGHT

I was always fascinated by Turkish delight as a kid. I don't even know if I liked the flavour, I just thought it was so unique and pretty. As an adult, I love these upgraded gelatin sweets, inspired by the flavours of traditional Turkish delight. Gelatin helps heal the gut lining and rose water is super calming for your belly, making these the perfect afternoon snack or evening sweet treat.

---

serving size depends on shape and cut

160ml pure pomegranate juice

85g raw honey

4 tablespoons powdered grass-fed gelatin

1 tablespoon rose water

A few pistachios, chopped (optional)

2–3 tablespoons arrowroot powder, for dusting (optional)

In a saucepan, combine the pomegranate juice, honey and 475ml water. Heat over medium heat until simmering.

In a small bowl, combine the gelatin and 60ml water and set aside for 5 minutes.

Stir the rose water into the pomegranate juice mixture. Add the gelatin mixture and stir well until the gelatin has dissolved. Remove from the heat and add the pistachios (if using).

Line a 20cm square glass baking dish with greaseproof paper, leaving about 3cm of overhang on all sides. Pour the mixture into the dish, cover and refrigerate for at least 3 hours, or overnight. Once set, cut it into rectangles or other shapes of your choice.

Spread the arrowroot powder in a deep dish and dust the pieces in the arrowroot to coat before serving.

Store in an airtight container in the fridge for up to 10 days.

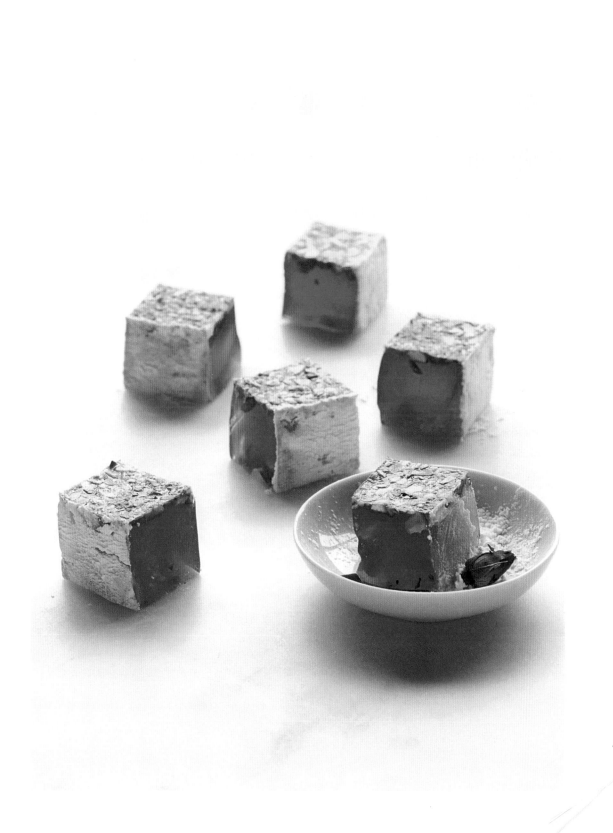

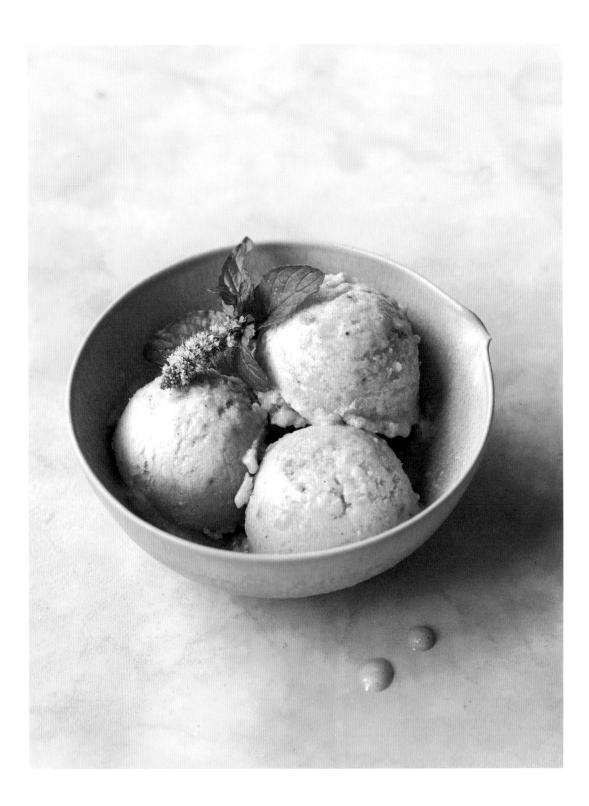

PEACHES 'N CREAM NICE CREAM

'Nice cream' is a standard warm-weather dessert in my household. I came up with this variation to highlight my daughter, Navy's, favourite summertime fruit. The addition of coconut milk and frozen banana adds the perfect amount of creaminess to the peaches. This recipe works well with any frozen fruit.

serves 2

450g frozen peaches

½ frozen ripe banana

80g coconut cream

½ teaspoon vanilla extract

Pinch of cinnamon

2 tablespoons collagen protein (optional)

Fresh mint, to decorate (optional)

Put all the ingredients except the mint into a high-speed blender or food-processor and process until smooth. (You may need to pulse a few times and scrape down the side.)

Divide between two small bowls, decorate with the mint, if you like, and enjoy immediately!

note

YOU CAN ALSO MAKE THIS NICE CREAM 'SCOOPABLE'. DOUBLE THE RECIPE AND POUR INTO A STANDARD LOAF TIN LINED WITH GREASEPROOF PAPER, THEN FREEZE FOR 2–3 HOURS OR OVERNIGHT SO IT HARDENS ENOUGH TO SCOOP WITH AN ICE CREAM SCOOPER.

SECRET

TRUFFLES

♢

Don't immediately turn the page when you see the first ingredient here – I promise these truffles do not taste a thing like beans! When blended well, black beans have a creamy texture that makes them a nice base for healthy truffles. When I have good chocolate around, I'll often eat most of the bar in one sitting, but with these truffles, I am able to have just two or three perfect bites and be good to go.

---

makes 10–15 truffles

1 x 400g tin black beans, drained and
   rinsed well

2 tablespoons pure maple syrup

3 tablespoons coconut oil

3 tablespoons unsweetened cocoa powder

2 tablespoons coconut butter

½ teaspoon pure vanilla extract

Pinch of sea salt

OPTIONAL TOPPINGS

Crushed pistachios

Unsweetened coconut flakes

Unsweetened cocoa powder

Sea salt

Toasted sesame seeds

Cayenne pepper

Combine all the truffle ingredients in a blender or food processor and blend until smooth.

Form truffles by rolling about 2 tablespoons of the mixture into balls with your hands and set them on a plate.

Roll the truffles in your choice of 'roll-in'.

Refrigerate at least 30 minutes before serving. Store in the fridge in an airtight container for up to one week, or in the freezer for up to one month.

tip

YOU CAN EXPERIMENT WITH ADDING THE
TOPPINGS DIRECTLY INTO THE TRUFFLE
MIXTURE, TOO!

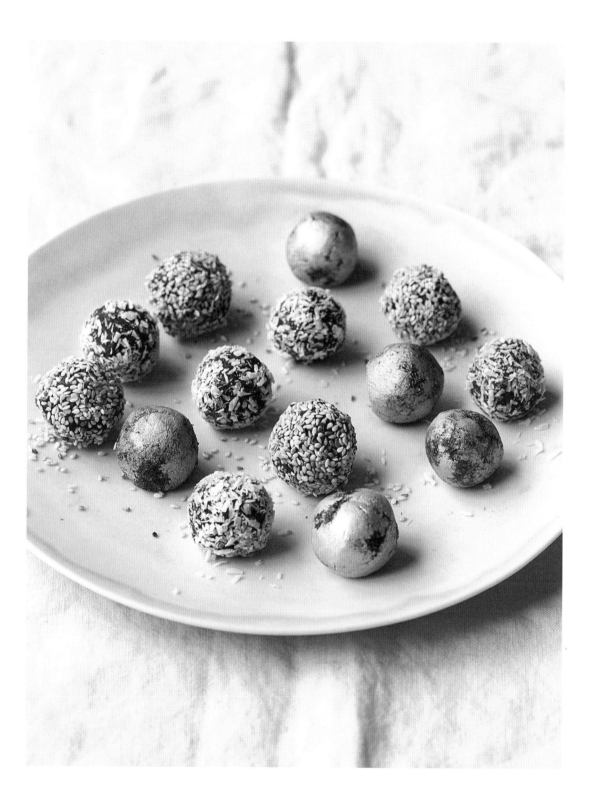

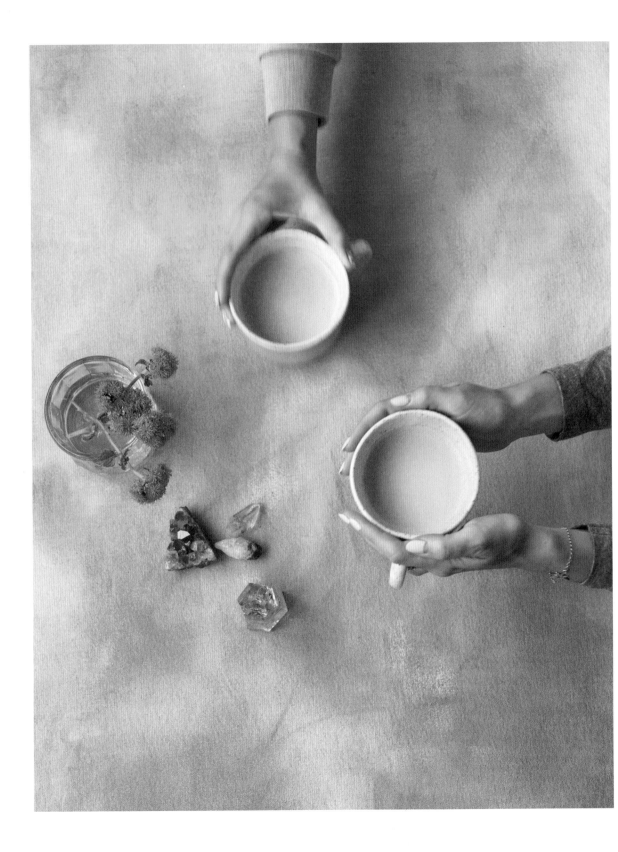

DRINKS

GO WITH YOUR GUT LEMONADE

◇

Back in the '90s, my mom was a Crystal Light lemonade queen and, truthfully, I loved it, too. This low-glycaemic, gut-friendly version is a refreshing alternative to both the Crystal Light of my youth and today's sugar or agave-loaded options. The cucumber and mint are soothing for your digestive system and the fennel gives this drink a fun flavour twist.

serves 1

½ small fennel bulb

1 lemon, peeled

1 Persian cucumber (or ½ larger cucumber, peeled)

Handful of fresh mint leaves

Liquid stevia (optional)

Combine the fennel, lemon, cucumber, mint and 475ml cold water in a high-speed blender and blend for 30 seconds. Pour through a fine-mesh strainer.

Taste and add more water or a drop or two of stevia, if wished.

variations

TRY USING SPARKLING WATER OR KOMBUCHA IN PLACE OF THE WATER. YOU CAN ALSO USE A JUICER (INSTEAD OF THE BLEND-AND-STRAIN PROCESS). IF YOU MAKE IT THIS WAY, TRY ADDING AN APPLE OR PEAR INSTEAD OF THE WATER AND OPTIONAL STEVIA.

FERMENTED FRUIT SODA

Kombucha is so last year... just kidding! But if you're looking for another cold, sweet and bubbly beverage to add to your gut-friendly toolkit, you'll want to try this easy-peasy ferment. Traditionally known as fruit kvass, this 'soda' is packed with good-for-your-gut probiotics and makes a great swap for traditional soda. Plus, kiddos of all ages love it too.

makes about 1 litre

Ripe fruit of choice (see note)
1 tablespoon raw honey
Filtered water

note

I TYPICALLY USE A MIX OF RASPBERRIES AND BLACKBERRIES BECAUSE THOSE ARE MY (AND NAVY'S) FAVOURITES, BUT FEEL FREE TO EXPERIMENT WITH ANYTHING THAT'S IN SEASON. USE ENOUGH FRUIT TO FILL THE JAR BY ONE THIRD TO HALF.

Place the fruit in a sterilised 2-litre preserving jar.

Mix the honey with a small amount of warm filtered water so it slightly dissolves and becomes less viscous.

Add the honey mixture to the jar and top up with filtered water, leaving some room at the top of the jar. Stir and seal tightly.

Set aside in a cool, dark place to ferment for 2–3 days, shaking the jar twice daily to prevent bacteria from forming on the surface. After 24 hours, you should see fermentation bubbles begin to appear. Taste your brew every day until you get that perfect mix of sweet and tangy that tastes best to you.

Strain the fruit soda (you can add the strained fruit to a smoothie for a probiotic fibre boost), transfer to a clean jar and store in the fridge for up to 2 weeks.

You can drink it straight (start with a small quantity, about 50ml) or you can add 1–2 tablespoons to your water throughout the day.

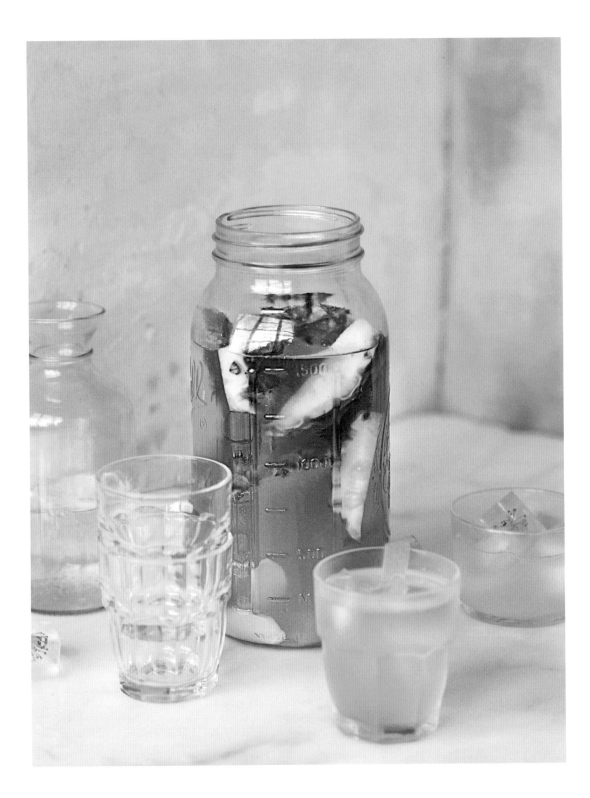

PINEAPPLE
TEPACHE

Hot summer days and nights call for cooling beverages – and if they can be of the fermented variety, even better! Pineapple tepache is essentially a fermented agua fresca, popular in Mexico and South America. This drink is lovely on its own but also makes a special base for upgraded cocktails – or mocktails.

makes about 8 cups

1 pineapple

75–150g coconut sugar, or other sweetener of choice

2–3cm piece of ginger, peeled and sliced

Filtered water

tip

MY FAVOURITE WAY TO ENJOY THIS DRINK IS TO USE IT TO FLAVOUR PLAIN SPARKLING WATER (AT A RATIO OF ABOUT 1 TO 3 TEPACHE TO WATER).

Rinse the pineapple lightly with water. You want to keep some of the natural yeasts that start the fermentation process. Cut the crown from the pineapple, then thickly cut off the peel so there is about 10–15mm of fruit left on the peel. Set the rest of the fruit aside to enjoy another time.

If you are using a granulated sweetener, first dissolve it in a small amount of hot water.

Place the pineapple peel and ginger in the bottom of a sterilised 2-litre jar. Add the sweetener to the jar and add filtered water to cover.

Weigh down the peels (you can do this with the crown of the pineapple) and cover the jar with a tea-towel or a piece of muslin, secured with a rubber band.

Set aside in a cool, dark place to ferment for 1–5 days, checking the flavour daily to achieve your desired taste. The longer you ferment it, the sourer and fizzier it will be.

When the tepache is fermented to your liking, strain it and serve over ice or store in a clean jar in the fridge for up to 2 weeks.

◇

MAGICAL
MORNING
MATCHA

This loaded matcha latte is deliciously frothy and gives a noticeable energy boost without the jitters and gut flare-ups that sometimes accompanies drinking regular coffee. Plus, it's a sweet vehicle for your current favourite superfoods and adaptogens – and looks great on your social media feed! Try this recipe, then post your Magical Morning Matcha to Instagram and tag me @RobynYoukilis and #YourHealthiestYou.

---

serves 1

475ml water, homemade hemp milk or a mix of the two

1 teaspoon ceremonial-grade matcha powder

1 tablespoon coconut butter (you can use ghee, but it will be a little less frothy)

2–4 tablespoons collagen powder

¼–½ teaspoon medicinal herbs, e.g. ashwagandha, rhodiola, or maca (I suggest no more than two at a time)

Bring the water to a near boil or bring the hemp milk (or hemp milk–water mixture) to a simmer in a small saucepan. Set aside to cool slightly, 3–5 minutes.

Combine the remaining ingredients in blender.

Add the water or hemp milk (or mixture) to the blender and blend for up to 1 minute.

Taste and adjust the ingredients if needed.

Pour, sip and enjoy!

tip

FOR EASY HOMEMADE HEMP MILK, BLEND 3 TABLESPOONS HEMP SEEDS AND 1 LITRE WATER

◇

THREE-SEED TEA

This traditional Ayurvedic tea is great for reducing bloating and inflammation in your digestive system. The combination of these three potent spices makes a healing tonic that's naturally caffeine-free so you can enjoy this soothing cup any time of day or night.

serves 5–6

1 teaspoon cumin seeds

1 teaspoon coriander seeds

1 teaspoon fennel seeds

Squeeze of fresh lemon or lime juice (optional)

Bring 1.2–1.4 litres of water to a boil in a small saucepan. Add the seeds and reduce the heat to maintain a simmer.

Simmer for 5–10 minutes, depending upon how strong you want the flavour.

Cool, then strain the liquid through a fine-mesh strainer into a glass jar or bottle. Add the lemon or lime juice, if using.

Drink 1 cup immediately and refrigerate the remainder to enjoy later.

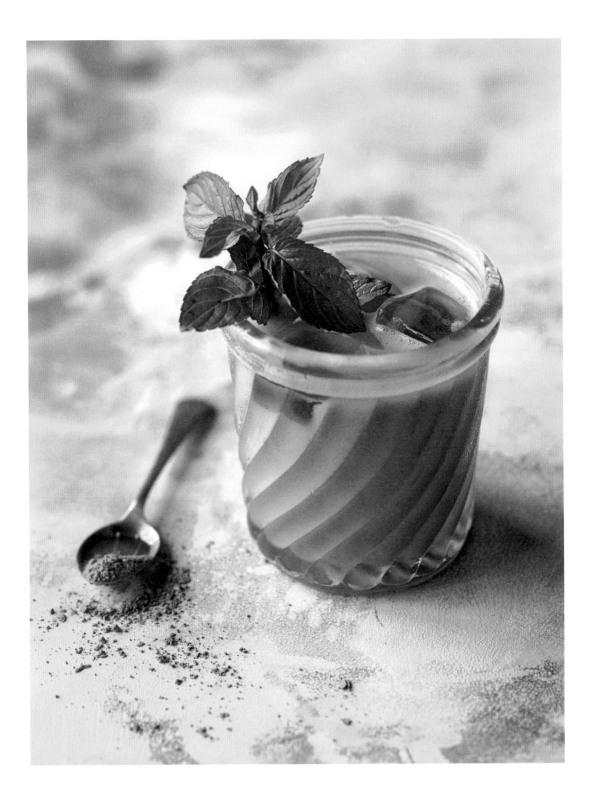

◇

CHOCO-MINT MATCHA LATTE

I discovered a rooftop herb garden on my building one evening while chasing a view of the sunset. And OMG, they had chocolate mint! The herb works perfectly here as it naturally lightens up traditionally earthy matcha in this fun variation of an iced tea latte. No chocolate mint? No problem. Regular mint and 1 teaspoon unsweetened cocoa powder will work just fine!

serves 1

120ml unsweetened vanilla milk alternative (I like almond or coconut here)

1 teaspoon ceremonial-grade matcha powder

A small handful of fresh chocolate mint leaves

tip

YOU CAN PURCHASE A HIGH-QUALITY 'INSTANT'-STYLE MATCHA THAT'S MEANT TO MIX DIRECTLY INTO COLD LIQUIDS. IF YOU'VE GOT THIS TYPE OF MATCHA, YOU CAN SIMPLY ADD ALL OF THE INGREDIENTS STRAIGHT INTO THE JAR, SEAL AND SHAKE (AND SKIP THE WHOLE FIRST STEP).

Heat the milk alternative to a low simmer in a small saucepan. Whisk in the matcha vigorously or blend in a high-speed blender.

Add the milk mixture, 240ml cold water, the mint leaves and a handful of ice cubes to a large preserving jar with a lid.

Seal and shake until well combined.

Add more ice cubes if needed, strain the mint and enjoy!

KOMBUCHA COCKTAIL

◇

The first bitters were created purely for medicinal purposes to help cure seasickness and stomach ailments. This cocktail incorporates digestion-friendly bitters and probiotic rich kombucha for a fun and healthy elixir. This cocktail is equally fabulous with or without the booze. Cheers!

serves 1

Ice

1 tablespoon fresh ginger juice

Juice of ½ lime

Juice of ½ lemon

40ml vodka (or additional kombucha if
   making mocktail version)

5 dashes of bitters

120ml kombucha

Twist of lemon or lime peel, to decorate
   (optional)

Half fill a cocktail shaker (or large preserving jar with lid) with ice. Add the ginger, lime and lemon juices, vodka and bitters and shake well.

Put the kombucha in a tall glass. Strain the vodka mixture over the kombucha.

Stir well and decorate with a twist of lemon or lime peel, if wished.

tip

YOU CAN MAKE GINGER JUICE WITHOUT A JUICER.
SIMPLY GRATE FRESH GINGER ROOT ON A MICROPLANE
GRATER AND SQUEEZE THE PULP TO EXTRACT THE JUICE.

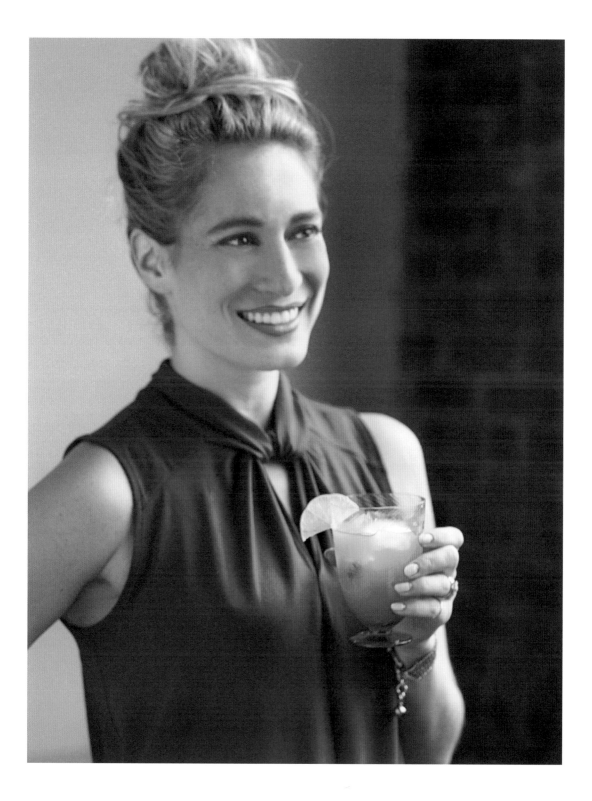

INDEX

THANK YOU!

From the bottom of my heart, thank you to every client, friend, teacher and moment of inspiration that made this book all that it is. To my book team, especially Kyle, Ellen, Nicky, and Gaby, for seeing my vision and bringing it to life. To my editor, Chris, for your hard work, humor, and flexibility with my usually missed deadlines. Thank you to my fabulous literary agents, Sarah and Celeste. Thank you Emily for your dedication and for making my work fun again. To my family, my nearest and dearest, especially my mama and brother. To my daughter, Navy, for giving me the gift of you, and the gift of finally feeling at peace in my body. And to my husband, Scott, thank you for supporting me body, mind and soul through this process. For stepping into our next level of us, and for reminding me that you like my tush, just the way it is.